Correctional Health Care Patient Safety Handbook

Reduce Clinical Error, Manage Risk, and Improve Quality

Correctional Health Care Patient Safety Handbook

*Reduce Clinical Error, Manage Risk,
and Improve Quality*

Lorry Schoenly
PhD, RN, CCHP-RN
Correctional Health Care Risk Consultant
Visiting Professor
Chamberlain College of Nursing
Graduate Nursing Program
Downers Grove, IL

Enchanted Mountain Press

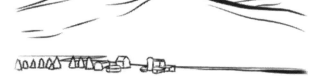

Published in the United States by Enchanted Mountain Press

ISBN: 978-0-9912942-1-3

Foreword

In the early nineteenth century, the French scholars Gustave de Beaumont and Alexis de Tocqueville examined prisons in the United States. Among other things, they described what they considered to be excessive punishment in some prisons, such as whipping prisoners at Sing Sing and Auburn penitentiaries in New York.[1] Since that time, our carceral system has both advanced and regressed. We continue to overuse segregation (isolation), as de Beaumont and de Tocqueville noted, and for the past forty years, U.S. public policy has promoted mass incarceration, with its attendant personal and social consequences.[2,3]

No longer permitted by law in the U.S., whipping is a punishment that is visible to the public eye. Cruelty, though, is not part of public policy. People are sentenced to prison *as* punishment, not *for* punishment. In the U.S., prisoners have a constitutional right to be free of cruel and unusual punishment.[4] This book is about prevention of the *in*visible punishment that can result from breaches in patient safety practices. It is a cogent primer on patient safety, through the lens of health care practices behind bars.

Correctional Health Care Patient Safety Handbook is a scholarly and practical guide for correctional health professionals to reduce the risk of unintentional harm to patients, harm that is often invisible to the public eye. This risk of harm is increased in an insular, command-control culture that sometimes has an unreasoning fear of change.

In the interests of our patients, our communities, and our fellow workers, we need to drive that change. Health care professionals have two primary duties: to prevent harm (non-maleficence) and to do good (beneficence). With this book, Lorry Schoenly provides clear direction toward preventing harm and thereby promoting health. This direction is soundly based on research and experience in the free-world health care community.

This book should be required reading for all health professionals working behind bars. Why? Because correctional health care is too often isolated from mainstream health care. As a result, practices behind bars do not always keep up. In the free-world community, patient safety practices have led to reduced morbidity and mortality. Correctional health professionals can use the same simple techniques toward the same end. Failure to do so can lead to pain and suffering (invisible to the public eye) and/or death.

Because of its isolation, correctional health care is often out of step with modern concepts in free-world health care, such as patient-centered care, primary care, prevention, and case management. This leads to breaches of continuity and coordination of care. The consequences can be barriers to timely access to an appropriate level of care. These are risky, from the points of view of the patient, the public health, and potential litigation.

The lessons in this volume on risk management, quality improvement, and patient safety are basic and critical to health workers' professionalism. Likewise, the lessons on teamwork, patient centeredness, avoiding error, acknowledging error, stereotyping avoidance and scope of practice are so very important to prudent and effective health care practices.

Most important, the use of the policies and practices described in this book will humanize health care behind bars. The last thing we want as health professionals is to be agents of pain. The end result will be improved professional satisfaction and better outcomes for our patients.

Robert B. Greifinger, MD

New York

May 2014

[1] Russell, Thomas. American Legal History-- Gustave de Beaumont & Alexis de Tocqueville, On the Penitentiary System in the United States and Its Application in France, (1833), accessed on April 30, 2014 at http://www.houseofrussell.com/legalhistory/alh/docs/penitentiary.html

[2] Travis, Jeremy. But They All Come Back, Urban Institute Press. Washington, DC (2005): xix-xx.

[3] Drucker, Ernest. A Plague of Prisons—the Epidemiology of Mass Incarceration in America

[4] Estelle v. Gamble, 429 U.S. 97 (1976); Farmer v. Brennan (92–7247), 511 U.S. 825 (1994)

Preface

Thank you for choosing to expand your understanding of patient safety and the application of safety principles in correctional health care. Even though patient safety has been a subject of great activity for decades in traditional settings, it is just emerging as a force in the specialized world of correctional health care.

How did you come to be concerned about patient safety? I must admit, like many in our specialty, my practice was molded by litigation concern and quality improvement efforts. As a nurse educator in a prison system of 26,000 incarcerated patients, I helped to implement clinical changes and develop staff competency to improve outcomes and reduce legal challenges. As I transitioned to consultation work I spent time helping jail and prison health care systems reduce risk by improving systems and processes. Several years back, while researching the literature to incorporate best practices into an evaluation tool, I made the link between patient safety and risk reduction. It was an "A-HA" moment that seems blatantly obvious as I recount it today. Yet, it took that moment for me to begin considering the vast literature on patient safety and how it might apply in the systems of care we use in the criminal justice system.

This book, then, is a culmination of my search for how to apply patient safety principles in correctional health care. Emanuel and colleagues (2008) provided the framework needed for the model that became the basis of this book. By organizing safety principles within categories of the environment, the systems, the patient, and the worker, we have a starting place for practical application in our setting. Here, then, in one resource, is a distillation of the current concepts of patient safety and the evidence-based practices that are in use in traditional health care settings with suggestions for how to apply these principles in correctional health care.

As I defend in the first chapter, patient safety is the appropriate motivator for risk reduction and quality improvement. Adopting a patient safety model reduces clinical error, manages risk, and improves quality – a triple-play of significant magnitude. I hope that you, too, will find that reframing your risk reduction and quality improvement efforts through a patient safety model will re-energize your clinical program and show significant results!

Lorry Schoenly, PhD, RN, CCHP-RN

Reviewers

Bruce P. Barnett, MD, JD, MBA
Past President, American Correctional
Health Services Association
CA/NV Chapter
Editor in Chief, CorHealth
Editorial Board Member, Journal of
Correctional Health Care
Sacramento, CA

Gayle F. Burrow, MPH, BSN, RN, CCHP-RN
Correctional Health Care Consultant
Maywood Park, OR

Robert B. Greifinger, MD
Correctional Health Care Consultant
New York, NY

Michelle Foster Earle, LNFA, ARM
President, OmniSure Consulting Group
Austin, TX

Rebekah Haggard, MD, CHCQM, CCHP
Vice President, Patient Safety Officer
Corizon
Nashville, TN

Catherine M. Knox, MN, RN, CCHP-RN
Correctional Health Care Consultant
Portland, OR

Johnnie R. Lambert, RN, CCHP
Licensed Healthcare Risk Manager
Vice-President, Policy and Accreditation
Clinical Operations
Armor Correctional Health Services, Inc.
Port Royal, SC

B. Sue Medley-Lane, RN, CCHP
Correctional Health Care Nurse
Consultant
Fort Lauderdale, FL

Kimberly M. Pearson, RN, MHA, MBA, CCHP
Deputy Agency Director – Correctional
Health Services
Orange County Health Care Agency
Santa Ana, CA

Sue Smith, RN, MSN, CCHP-RN
Correctional Nurse Educator
Ashville, OH

Marc F. Stern, MD, MPH
Correctional Health Care Consultant
Seattle, WA

Kathryn J. Wild, RN, MPA, CCHP
Correctional Health Care Consultant
Retired Director of Correctional Health
San Bernardino & Orange County, CA

Acknowledgement

Neither nurses nor authors work in isolation; thus, as a nurse author, I have many people to thank for their contributions to this text. Writing can seem an isolating activity, but my Facebook and Twitter tribes kept me sane and motivated. Many thanks to my friends and followers who frequently kept me from hitting the delete button and tossing my keyboard through the window.

My most significant cheerleader, though, is my husband and lifelong friend, Walt Schoenly. Although the closest he gets to our world is through table talk and an occasional Lockup episode, he was always willing to provide wise direction and lighten my mood when the words were flowing like sludge and the muses were out playing in another sandbox.

Book reviewers are the lifeblood in any good text. This book's reviewers provided the practical insight to make this book a helpful guide. Special thanks to Robert Greifinger, Catherine Knox, and Marc Stern, who were willing to read the entire manuscript and point out areas of incongruity or incomprehensibility.

Finally, I am thankful for you, the reader, who obviously wants to improve the health care delivered to our vulnerable and disadvantaged patients. You have motivated me to write this book!

Contents

1 Risk Management, Quality Improvement, and Patient Safety

Attention to professional liability issues is critical in correctional health care. With easy access to the court system, the inmate patient population is often quick to bring suit alleging wrongful treatment. While medical malpractice claims seem to be decreasing in traditional settings (Rothstein, 2010), concern about correctional health care claims remains high. Although no specific national database for corrections claims is available, the Massachusetts Correctional Legal Services have identified health care as the most common issue that prisoners raise for seeking their legal assistance (Thompson, 2010).

The foundation for constitutional litigation regarding medical care behind bars was laid by a 1976 Supreme Court decision (Greifinger, 2007). *Estelle v Gamble* established timely access to an appropriate level of health care as a right of every prisoner and deemed the withholding of health care cruel and unusual punishment as defined by the 8th (and the 14th in the case of pre-trial detainees) amendment to the US Constitution. Legal precedent and civil law over the next three decades created a health care system whose structure is often based on legal requirement rather than patient benefit. Since 1976, correctional health care practice has been molded by case law, court order, or consent decree (Rold, 2007). This led to a legally-focused risk management system as those providing health care in the criminal justice system must be attuned to both civil rights and malpractice legal concerns.

Traditional health care settings have also focused on reducing legal liability, but have used a dual system for responding to legal concerns. Liability is reduced through risk management programs while continuous quality improvement programs were developed to respond to clinical quality issues. The recent push toward patient safety in the wake of the 1999 Institute of Medicine's publication of *To Err is Human: Building a Safer Health System* (2000) has led to the consideration of a third, and improved, option: a focus not on institutional or caregiver concerns but on the patient's safety - thus centering on doing less harm. Focusing on patient safety can reduce legal liability and improve clinical quality.

Organizing health care processes around patient safety can be particularly helpful in a setting such as correctional health care. The fragmented nature of care delivery, the transient nature of the patient population, and the added application of security structures can overwhelm and overshadow patient care.

Differentiating Risk Management, Quality Improvement, and Patient Safety Frameworks

Risk management, quality improvement, and patient safety efforts ultimately affect clinical error, but each has a different focus. Table 1.1 differentiates the focus and components of these three frameworks. Each of these are often managed by different parts of the organization with little communication, integration, or collaboration (ECRI Institute, 2009), resulting in weak and ineffective outcomes.

Table 1.1. Differentiation of Risk Management, Quality Improvement and Patient Safety

Program	Risk Management	Quality Improvement	Patient Safety
Focus	Reduce/prevent financial Loss	Improve processes and outcomes of patient care	Prevent patient harm
Locus of Management	Finance	Management	Clinical
Processes	• Claims management • Contract/policy review • Regulatory and accreditation compliance	• Benchmarking • Best practices/clinical guidelines • Improvement projects	• Clinical process change • Systems thinking • Simplification, standardization and "built-in" reliability processes
Outcomes	Reduced financial loss	Efficient and effective clinical program	Reduced clinical error

Information from ECRI Institute, 2009; Napier & Youngberg, 2011; Wachter, 2012

Risk Management

Risk is defined as a chance of loss. The purpose of a risk management program is to "protect the organization against risks associated with accidental losses, regardless of the cause" (McCaffrey & Hagg-Rickert, 2009, p.8). This focus is, by definition, on the organization primarily with a financial direction and motivation. Risk managers monitor and intervene to prevent and reduce loss in areas of patient care, medical staff, employees, property, and financial risk. The risk management process involves identifying and analyzing loss exposures in order to implement necessary changes to reduce further exposure. A risk management program can encompass claims management, contract and policy review, and regulatory and accreditation compliance functions (Napier & Youngberg, 2011). When performed correctly, risk management successfully reduces financial loss to a health care organization. A secondary result is often the reduction of clinical error.

Quality Improvement

Health care quality assurance programs began in the 1980s with the Joint Commission's quality assurance standards that required hospital systems to establish a formal program for monitoring care delivery (ECRI Institute, 2009). Quality assurance methods gave way to quality improvement, as methodology from industry and technology was applied in the health care setting. For example, the popular health care quality improvement model "PDSA" (Plan, Do, Study, Act) was first developed for industry by statistician W. Edward Deming (Moen & Norman, 2011). Standards for quality improvement also made their way into correctional health care and both major accreditation bodies – the National Commission on Correctional Health Care (NCCHC) and the American Correctional Association (ACA) – have quality improvement requirements (NCCHC, 2014; ACA, 2010).

Quality improvement activities to improve the efficiency and effectiveness of patient care are typically included as part of a clinical manager's job functions. Improvement projects are selected based on determination of ineffective or inefficient care processes; these may be decided through benchmarking and best practice determinations. Successful quality improvement initiatives produce change that results in a more effective and efficient clinical program. As with risk management, reducing clinical error is often a welcome by-product.

Patient Safety

The primary goal of patient safety is to do less harm during the delivery of necessary health care. This emerging discipline focuses on clinical systems and the interaction of caregivers operating within the systems to "minimize the incidence and impact of, and maximize recovery from, adverse events" (Emanuel et al., 2008, p.1). Adverse events are defined as any injury caused by medical care, although Wachter (2012) points out that adverse events may not be caused by error but may result from the underlying disease process or an aspect of the diagnosis or treatment of a condition. Patient safety programs, however, focus primarily on clinical error reduction, as nearly 80,000 annual patient deaths have been directly linked to clinical error (Reed & May, 2011). Patient safety, then, is a clinical process (rather than a financial or management process) that involves regular evaluation and revision of the clinical program to reduce error through simplification, standardization, and introduction of redundancy (Dekker, 2011). Effective patient safety measures reduce clinical error – a leading cause of patient litigation. As such, an argument can be made that patient safety is *the primary component* of risk management. A patient safety perspective also makes sense for continuous quality improvement as this focus also results in improvement of processes and outcomes of patient care.

A Patient Safety Model for Correctional Health Care

A patient safety model for health care proposed by Emanuel et al. (2008) involves the interaction of the recipients of care, the systems for therapeutic action and the health care workers. Surrounding this interaction is the environment of care, which is critical when providing care in the correctional setting. Thus, these four domains encompass the various principles of patient safety and provide an organ-izing framework for applying patient safety principles to actual practice in the correctional setting (Figure 1.1). The domains of environment, systems, patients and workers are briefly described here and will be individually explored in future chapters.

Figure 1.1 A Patient Safety Model of Health Care

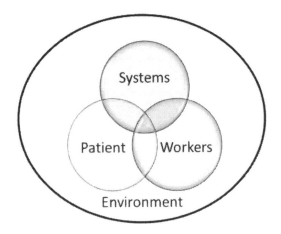

Adapted from Emanuel et al., 2008

Environment of Care

The environment in which health care is provided affects the interaction of the patient, the health care workers, and the systems used to deliver care. The environment is primarily the organizational culture of the workplace but can also include the physical environment such as the design of the care delivery setting and the available equipment and supplies. The secure environment of the criminal justice system adds intensity to the environment of care by also imparting a unique set of values and cultural norms. A patient safety framework seeks to advance the organization to a Just Culture that is continually learning and improving. Components of the Environment of Care domain are discussed in Chapter 2.

Systems for Therapeutic Action

Patient care is delivered through a complex system of intertwined processes. The patient and health care workers interact with these systems of therapeutic action within the environment of care. Patient safety principles can increase the reliability of care systems, reducing error and improving outcomes. Components of the Systems for Therapeutic Action domain are discussed in Chapter 3.

Patient-Recipient of Care

The patient, as recipient of care, is also a vital part of the safety framework. Interacting with health care workers and the systems of therapeutic action within the environment of care, patients have opportunity to actively participate in and monitor care delivery. There are many barriers to engaging patients in the criminal justice system that must be considered and overcome. Components of the Recipient of Care domain are discussed in Chapter 4.

Health Care Workers

The competence and judgment of health care staff is a major factor in patient safety. Staff interact with the patient and take therapeutic actions to deliver health care. Internal and external factors such as fatigue, work stress, impairment and shift rotation affect worker's abilities to deliver safe care. Components of the Health Care Worker domain are discussed in Chapter 5.

Five Principles of Patient Safety

Five key principles that underlie a patient safety program are a Just Culture in a learning organization, high reliability systems design, communication and teamwork, patient-centered care, and competent care providers (Dekker, 2011; Spath, 2011; Wachter, 2012). These principles can be organized within the four domains in the proposed model of patient safety (Table 1.2) and will provide structure to discuss each patient safety domain in future chapters.

A Just Culture in a Learning Organization

An organization's culture is the shared beliefs and meaning of actions that are pervasive among the individuals working within the environment. This culture can be determined by the common attitudes and meanings given to staff actions and the outcomes of those actions. A culture of safety, then, involves shared beliefs among the members that enhance patient safety. Elements of organizational culture found to enhance patient safety include respect and civility, a regard for safety as a top priority, enhanced teamwork and collaboration among all disciplines and levels in the organization, and openness and transparency about

Table 1.2. Domains and Principles of Patient Safety

Domain of Patient Safety	Principle of Patient Safety
Environment of Care	A Just Culture in a Learning Organization
Systems for Therapeutic Action	High Reliability System Design Communication and Teamwork
Recipient of Care	Patient-Centered Care
Health Care Workers	Competent Care Providers

clinical errors when they take place (Barnsteiner, 2012). The willingness to report clinical error is based on an organizational understanding of the causes of error, as well as the interplay of the environment, clinical systems, health care workers and care recipients. A safety culture seeks to discover and correct flaws in the system. A Just Culture adds individual practitioner accountability to the concept of safety in an organization's culture (Burhans, Chastain, & George, 2012).

In a Just Culture, system design issues are balanced with individual accountability in evaluating a clinical error. It shifts the focus from that of errors and outcomes to one of system design and behavioral choices. This can be a huge culture change from that of blame and punishment that is sometimes found in a correctional setting. When health care staff have a real fear of being escorted out of the building for a clinical error, reporting near-miss and clinical mistakes is severely hampered.

A Just Culture is enhanced by a management philosophy that emphasizes ongoing staff development and system changes based on continuous learning about how the organization operates (Finkelman, 2009). Engaging in organizational learning requires openness, honesty and trust among peers throughout all levels of the organization. Punitive, blaming cultures are unwilling to learn from failure. They are unable to uncover and communicate about the causes of clinical error, thus missing the lessons to be learned (Edmondson, 2004). Organizational learning is movement toward a common goal – such as safer patient care – by adapting and changing the organization based on the collective experience. As it relates to clinical errors, a learning organization extracts meaningful lessons from adverse or near-miss events and converts these lessons into improvements in structures and processes (Dekker, 2011).

High Reliability System Design

High reliability is critical in any system with increased likelihood of catastrophic events. High reliability system design first emerged in the nuclear power and air traffic control industries, where error can result in the significant loss of life. Since the emergence of data on the high number of deaths in health care related to clinical error, these design principles are increasingly applied in the clinical setting with positive result. High reliability design establishes system defenses to avoid human error (Reason, 2000). Safeguards and barriers within the care delivery system are a primary means of error prevention.

Re-engineering clinical processes using high reliability principles involves seeking system changes that reduce human error. Concepts of high reliability design include mindfulness of potential error, formal structures and procedures that incorporate redundancy checks, and an informal culture open to safety accountability at all levels of the organization (Carroll & Rudolph, 2006). Common tools used in high reliability systems include buffers to detect error before it reaches the patient, reminders to help avoid reliance on memory, forced functions such as requiring specific actions before allowing movement to a next process step, and constraints within a process (Spath, 2011).

Decentralized decision-making authority for safety processes is a key component of high reliability system design (Dekker, 2011). Correctional settings, however, typically rely on a centralized command-and-control structure that may not value front-line innovation. Even in these situations, staff must be encouraged to suggest system changes to improve patient safety, as they have a unique perspective on successful day-to-day health care operations.

Health care systems are complex adaptive systems where the communication among the parts is as important as the parts themselves (Wachter, 2012). This is particularly true in a correctional setting where there is an added layer of communication with security officers, custody administration and, in jail settings, the police as well. The interaction of multiple decision-makers increases the need for a high reliability system design.

Communication and Teamwork

Communication is identified as a top reason for clinical error. In fact, 80% of clinical errors can be traced to miscommunication (The Joint Commission, 2012). The safe delivery of patient care requires a written and oral communication structure, solid processes for hand-off of patient care, and open communication of patient care concerns among the team members. Patient care is not accomplished in isolation, although many of the health care disciplines are trained in educational systems emphasizing individual practice. Without effective systems of communication or the appropriate use of them, patient information can be lost, care can be diminished or treatments can be inappropriately applied.

Effective communication and teamwork in the correctional setting must overcome barriers imposed by security requirements. For example, health care staff may need to negotiate timing or location of care delivery with security officers, adding an additional layer of collaborative work. When the goals of health care and security conflict, tension builds, resulting in communication breakdown. Organizational structure can create communication silos that hinder safe patient care. Staff on off-shifts may need to communicate about patients with covering providers who are not familiar with the patient or the correctional environment. Many diagnostics and treatments must be accomplished outside the security perimeter. Communication with laboratories, diagnostic centers and specialty services can falter without well-established communication systems and astute, accountable practitioners.

For many reasons, often financial, correctional settings have been slower than their counterparts in other health care settings to adopt electronic medical records (EMRs). Unfortunately, written documentation in medical records increases the chances of miscommunication through poor handwriting, missing reports or inaccessible records at the point of care delivery. EMRs are not without their safety issues, however, as human error can still lead to missing or incorrect data and technical failures (Sparnon & Marella, 2012). EMRs created for traditional health care settings are often difficult to adapt to the unique clinical processes of corrections.

Patient-Centered Care

A patient-centered approach to care mitigates against the fragmented care delivery system inherent in the correctional environment. A patient focus – rather than an organizational or caregiver focus – shifts care-delivery priorities toward decreasing patient harm. The Institutes of Medicine (IOM, 2001) defines patient-centered care as "providing care that is respectful of and responsive to individual patient preferences, needs, and values and ensuring that patient values guide all clinical decisions" (p. 6). This is a tall order in the correctional environment, where individualized attention may conflict with a system that values anonymity and no-one is allowed to receive specialized service or care. Yet, the patient is a key component of safety in the complex health care system: an active and informed patient provides additional safeguards and redundancy in care delivery. For example, patients can help with the prevention and early detection of potential error (Aspden & IOM, 2004).

Competent Care Providers

Recruiting, selecting, and hiring competent care providers are important components of safe health care delivery. This requires time and expertise, which can be lacking in a correctional health system. Although the last few decades have ushered in major improvements in this regard, the correctional setting can still be viewed as a refuge for poor practitioners. In order to continue improvements, unsafe practitioners should be eliminated from the system.

Correctional health systems are challenged to provide the time and finances to adequately orient newly-hired staff and maintain the competence of incumbent staff. Staff development activities are rarely handled by dedicated staff educators and more likely considered a part of a unit manager's responsibilities along with financial, staffing, and clinical responsibilities. New staff may be unfamiliar with the unique nature of the secure environment and the inmate population. They must quickly learn to negotiate both the health care and the custody hierarchies to safely accomplish care. The autonomous nature of delivering health care in correctional environments requires staff members to fully understand the limits of their licensure and job descriptions. Strict boundaries, identified in a traditional health care setting by policies, procedures, and organizational accountability structures, may be missing in the correctional setting. The uninformed health care professional can easily be swayed into inappropriate action by assuming that "it must be safe" if the request was made by a person of authority in the organization.

Patient Safety Principles Applied in the Correctional Setting

Patient safety principles advocated in traditional settings require practical translation to the criminal justice environment and the unique characteristics of the patient population. The National Commission on Correctional Health Care accreditation standards include a patient safety standard which emphasizes the implementation of patient safety systems to prevent adverse and near-miss clinical events, voluntary reporting of adverse and near-miss events in a non-punitive environment, as well as methods for the organization to evaluate and learn from clinical errors that take place (NCCHC, 2014).

Experts from both the public and private sector collaborated to create a list of patient safety standards for correctional health care (Stern, Greifinger, & Mellow, 2010). Seven categories of patient safety measures are proposed:

- Access to and availability of care

- Culture of safety

- Personnel

- Medical management

- Transitions and communication

- Patient involvement

- Specific condition

These standards have stimulated continued discussion about patient safety in the correctional environment and fit within the four domains of the Patient Safety Model described more fully in succeeding chapters (Table 1.3).

Table 1.3. The Patient Safety Model and Proposed Correctional Health Care Safety Standards

Model Domain	Correctional Health Care Safety Standards
Environment of Care	Culture of Safety
Systems for Therapeutic Action	Access to and Availability of Care Medical Management Transitions and Communication Special Conditions
Recipient of Care	Patient Involvement
Health Care Workers	Personnel

Models of Error Causation

Understanding the causes of clinical error when conducting system evaluation and improvement will significantly improve patient safety. Here again, the application of principles forged in other industries can accelerate safety improvements in health care. Several models of error causation provide a holistic approach to error analysis, organizational action, and error prevention.

Active and Latent Failures

Clinical errors usually have many attributing causes, which are categorized as either active or latent failures. Active failures are those readily apparent causes that can be seen at the point of care (Wachter, 2012). These are most often the actions taken by a care provider, such as the example of a nurse giving a patient the wrong dose of a medication due to a mathematical error. Latent failures, on the other hand, are less obvious system design flaws. These are embedded in the system, often invisible at the point of care (Henriksen, Dayton, Keyes, Carayon, & Hughes, 2008). In the aforementioned wrong dose example, the error may have also been caused by a lack of unit dosing in the pharmaceutical operations and short-staffing that led to this nurse working a double shift.

Blunt End and Sharp End of Clinical Error

Viewing a clinical error from the "blunt end" and "sharp end" of care delivery can also be helpful (Figure 1.2). The blunt end, upstream from the clinical error, involves the many complexities of the structure and process in health care delivery that influence the point of care but are removed from it (Wachter, 2012). This corresponds to latent system failures. Examples might be staffing patterns, a culture of silence, or poor training resources for off-shift staff. The sharp end of clinical error is the point of patient contact; it corresponds with active system failures. In the prior wrong dose example, the sharp end of the clinical error involved the nurse's dose miscalculation and the administration of the medication.

Figure 1.2 Blunt End/Sharp End of Clinical Error

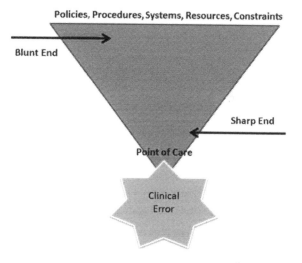

Adapted from Carroll, 2009

Swiss Cheese Model of Clinical Error

This helpful model developed by Reason (2000) uses the image of the many and varied holes in Swiss cheese as an analogy for the safety gaps in error protection that are incorporated into health care processes (Figure 1.3). This model proposes that a clinical error happens when multiple "holes" line up in the layers of system protection to allow penetration of the safety system and result in harm. Layers in the system may include various components of both the blunt end and the sharp end of the patient care system, and involve both active and latent failures.

Analyzing the wrong dose medication error using this model might identify causation through inappropriate pharmacy ordering practices, incomplete staff orientation and inadequate staffing to initiate a double-check process for the high-alert medication list. In the correctional setting, issues with security interface, the geography of care settings within the facility, and characteristics of the patient population can add additional layers to further complicate the process.

All modern models of error causation take a systems approach – rather than a person approach – to clinical error. A person approach focuses solely on the sharp end of the process and assumes that primary responsibility rests on the individual provider at the point of care. In the person approach, error is the result of forgetfulness, inattention, carelessness or negligence (Reason, 2000). Research on

Figure 1.3 Swiss Cheese Model of Clinical Error

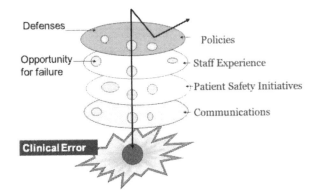

Adapted from Reason, 2000

error reduction has shown that, although the provider needs to be a part of the equation, a majority of the causes of error are inherent within the health care system (Dekker, 2011; Spath, 2011; Wachter, 2012). Changes to the system that reduce error achieve the greatest results.

Human Factors Engineering

Research into the human factors causing error in other industries also provides a model of causation that has been applied successfully in health care settings. Human factors engineering concepts can assist providers in determining how to best go about improving a failure-prone system or process. Spath (2011) suggests the following remedies for human factors in error causation:

- Reducing reliance on memory, such as the use of checklists;

- Improving information access, as when protocols are readily available to a provider at the point of care;

- Mistake-proofing processes, as when a medication dispensing system will not allow access without entering the patient's identification;

- Standardizing tasks, such as withdrawal monitoring; and

- Reducing the number of hand-offs, as in maintaining the same provider group for the on-call schedule.

Normalization of Deviance

In a complex system involving many staff members, various equipment failures, and communication challenges, deviation from protocol can become normalized. The term "normalization of deviance" was first coined during the investigation of the fatal Shuttle Challenger disaster in 1986. Inquiry revealed cases of overlooked warnings such as inclement weather forecasts and prior O-ring (a mechanical gasket) concerns. Since previous instances of these deviations did not result in injury, they were treated as normal and were not fully included in the launch decision. By cutting corners, ignoring protocol, repeatedly silencing equipment alarms, and disregarding standard safety checks, deviation is normalized and becomes standard protocol in a health care setting (Wachter, 2012).

Secondary to normalization of deviance is the establishment of a "culture of low expectation." This culture develops in a setting where team members begin to anticipate faulty behavior and incomplete communication. Instead of demanding safe procedure, participants grow accustomed to the mediocre culture and participate in it (Chassin & Becher, 2002). A culture of low expectation combined with normalization of deviance further increases the risk of clinical error and patient injury.

A Correctional Health Care Risk Reduction Program

Patient safety is foundational to a successful risk reduction program and provides support for every program component. Risk reduction in correctional health care includes both traditional processes and elements that are unique to the practice setting – in particular, the inmate grievance process, civil rights issues related to claims, the involvement of security personnel, and the communication systems within a secure environment.

Adverse Event Analysis

An adverse event is any injury caused by medical care. Adverse event analysis proactively identifies and corrects potential system failures (Spath, 2011). Adverse event analysis differentiates clinical error from other types of injury and seeks to prevent similar errors from arising in the future. The components of adverse event analysis are identification, cumulative tracking, and evaluation.

Identification. A solid system of adverse event analysis starts with event identification. Under-reporting of adverse events is well-established in health care, with estimates as high as 96% unreported (Dekker, 2011). Some adverse events are public and easily identified; however, many more clinical errors are hidden from view and require self-reporting to initiate reflection and action. Establishing mechanisms for reporting adverse events, then, is a necessary process for risk reduction.

Most health care organizations have some form of error reporting; often, this is a simple report form for a medication or treatment error. Sometimes, an incident report form is used to document a real or potential clinical error situation. How effectively the system is activated, however, is better determined by how the information is used once a form is submitted, rather than the organization of the form or process. A Just Culture improves the likelihood of reporting an adverse or near-miss event. A culture of blame, humiliation or retaliation will prevent honest declaration and thoughtful reflection on clinical error, without which patient safety is difficult (Aspden & IOM, 2004).

For adverse event identification to effectively enhance organizational learning and reduce future error, institutions must be attuned to the structure and process of initial event reporting. First, the reporting of errors must be non-punitive, protected, and voluntary (Dekker, 2011). This is especially true for errors that might have been caused by a significant breach in protocol; however, any error reporting can be mishandled in a dysfunctional or punitive environment. Staff members must feel that the information they share will be handled fairly and treated confidentially. Many systems are based on staff reporting adverse events to first-line managers. Other systems have error reporting processed through a line position such as a risk manager. Staff perception about the use of the information provided underlies the degree of error reporting in any organization (Wachter, 2012).

The format of the written report is an important structural component of adverse event reporting. Many settings use a forced-choice format in which the initiator checks off boxes categorized by the type of error and level of harm. While indexing in this manner helps create quantitative reports for trending and for determination of organizational concern, it requires the initiator to evaluate the event prematurely. Many events are multi-faceted and multi-causal. Those practicing at the sharp end of the care delivery system may not adequately consider causes arising from the blunt end of the system. In addition, harm may be hard to quantify initially. The forced-choice format can lead to under- or over-estimation of the cause(s) of error.

Error causation stripped of context in an indexing reporting system reduces organizational learning as well as future patient harm reduction. The "story" of the incident provides clues to the panoply of causes to be considered in the investigation process (Dekker, 2011), but forced-choice reporting requires the initiator to strip out story and context in order to make determinations about the event that fit the category options on the form. A robust adverse event reporting system takes into account both the quantitative and qualitative elements of the event.

A final issue for consideration in creating an effective adverse event reporting system is determining what events rise to the level necessary for reporting. This may, in fact, be the crux of the issue in many settings. If every error or potential error requires reporting, there is little likelihood of being able to differentiate a signal among the noise (Dekker, 2011). It is often by experience that a health care provider determines that a situation is important to report. This experience must also be balanced with a healthy concern for a normalization of deviance (described in the prior causation section). For example, if a medication is administered late due to a security delay in initiating pill line, is that worthy of reporting? What determines the seriousness of the "wrong time" medication error? Does the practitioner need to evaluate the patient's disease state and treatment regimen? What if this delay happens several times each week? Systems must weigh such issues and provide guidance to staff about what constitutes a reportable error.

> "Every adverse event should be a learning event. By nature, the review process is retrospective and thus hindsight bias cannot be avoided. Many times we hear the push-back or complaint that event review is just 'Monday morning quarterbacking' - but what do great quarterbacks do on Monday morning? Quarterbacks watch film to search for opportunities to improve their pass, to raise their awareness for defensive moves and to find the passing lane for a touchdown next game. Likewise, the goal of adverse event review is to learn as much as possible about what happened, why and how to mitigate future recurrences. So yes, it does involve 'Monday morning quarterbacking' and there will be no apologies for 'studying film' to improve our care and enhance patient safety"
> – **Rebekah Haggard, MD, CHCQM, CCHP, Vice President and Patient Safety Officer, Corizon, Nashville, TN**

Cumulative tracking. Although each adverse event must be evaluated individually, cumulative tracking of types of events provides important systems information. Here is where efforts to quantify types of events can be important. Cumulative tracking helps identify persistent systems issues and failure-prone processes that must be addressed. Quantification can also determine priorities for system changes. A consistent method for accumulating and reporting adverse events is an important component of both risk management and quality improvement efforts.

Evaluation. The power of an adverse event reporting program is in the evaluation process. Evaluation takes into consideration elements of error causation including active/latent, blunt end/sharp end, and gaps in safety mechanisms when the "holes" in the Swiss cheese align. Adverse event evaluation then considers engineering human factors concepts and potential for normalization of deviation in determining a course of action to reduce likelihood of another such event.

Root Cause Analysis

A primary mode of adverse event evaluation is root cause analysis, which reconstructs the events and trajectory of an incident to determine causative factors and safety failure modes. The strength of root cause analysis is the ability to thoroughly evaluate all possible contributing causes for the event, rather than simply relying on the first or most obvious cause discovered on investigation (Wachter, 2012). The root cause analysis process involves asking three primary questions about the event:

1. What happened?

2. Why did it happen?

3. What can be done to prevent it from happening again? (Department of Veterans Affairs National Center for Patient Safety, 2009)

Systematically answering these questions can reveal latent and active components of an incident so that evaluators are able to develop a more accurate picture of the context of a clinical error. The "Why" question should be asked multiple times to dig deeper into causality. For example, failure to notify the provider about a critical lab value which results in a patient injury may, at first, seem to be a communication error on the part of the laboratory service. Asking the "Why" question successively, it is found that the laboratory automatically faxes critical values to the site. The fax machine is located in the health service administrator's office, which is locked and unattended on Saturdays, the day of the event. Per protocol, the laboratory service also calls the phone of the ordering physician. The physician in this example does not carry his work cell phone when not on-call, and the on-call physician for that weekend uses a different cell phone number posted for weekend staff but not available to the laboratory service.

Factors contributing to adverse events. Developing an effective root cause analysis requires a determination of all possible factors contributing to adverse events in the clinical setting. Henriksen et al. (2008) provides a thorough framework for determining contributing factors, from latent conditions to active errors (Figure 1.4). This five-tier framework is appropriate for correctional health care programs to use in evaluating adverse events. When using the framework to

Figure 1.4 Contributing Factors for Adverse Events in Health Care

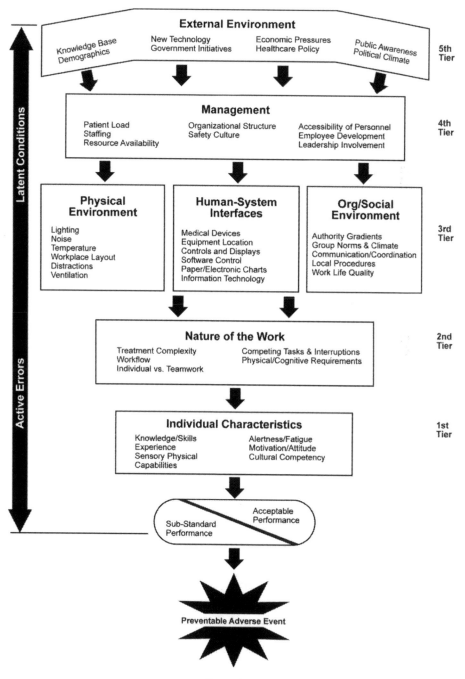

From Henriksen et al., 2008, pg.7. Public Domain.

evaluate causation, begin with the first tier (closest to the patient) and move outward, considering the contribution of each tier to the resulting event. Latent conditions that may be hidden from view in the initial evaluation become visible. System change is necessary when a latent issue emerges regularly in the root cause analysis of individual adverse events. For example, if staff fatigue is implicated in a first-tier evaluation of several events, additional consideration can be given to patient load and staffing conditions in the fourth-tier evaluation of the events.

"How" and "Why" questions guide a root cause analysis through the various tiers of contributing factors. In the initial round of evaluation, this is an educated guess on the part of the investigation team. Validation of the resulting hypotheses then determines the next course of action. The team may find that they must search further back in the sequence of events for latent causes not apparent in the initial resulting error evaluation (Spath, 2011). A rich field of inquiry is produced from a thorough root cause analysis of a single significant adverse event or multiple similar events that might suggest a system failure.

The investigators must determine all possible causes of a clinical error in order to create a plan of action. Active causes are easier to correct than latent causes, and, therefore, it can be tempting to primarily focus on correction of active causes. Latent cause correction, however, will result in more significant harm reduction organization-wide because these causes, at the blunt end of care delivery, affect multiple aspects of care.

Avoiding error in determining causation. Mental tendencies and personal preferences can invade the adverse event analysis and require vigilance to prevent or eliminate. Three common evaluation biases are of particular concern:

- *Hindsight bias* results when investigators look back on a situation with the knowledge of the outcome. From this vantage point, the error trajectory is clearly visible and assumed to be clearly visible to the individuals at the point of care. However, at the time of the actual event, multiple variables were vying for the individual's attention and judgment, making the future outcome less apparent (Murphy, Shannon, & Pugliese, 2009).

- *Attribution error bias* pins a clinical error on a character flaw or defect in the individual at the sharp end of care delivery. An attribution error bias would likely settle primary blame for a clinical error on the negligence or incompetence of the staff involved rather than seek full understanding of the system issues contributing to the event (Henriksen et al., 2008).

- *Confirmation bias* is a tendency to accept evidence that supports a favored working hypothesis (Wachter, 2012). Hindsight bias and attribution error bias can contribute to confirmation bias. In an environment that seeks out individuals to blame, confirmation bias would encourage investigators to stop seeking causation once individual error is identified.

Adverse event analysis is a primary function of risk management. A structure that supports patient safety principles in reporting and analyzing adverse events will also support the reduction of patient harm and liability in the correctional setting.

Inmate Grievance Management

Management of inmate grievances is another key component of risk management in correctional health care. An inmate grievance is equivalent to a patient complaint in a traditional health care setting. Grievances can involve a variety of situations and conditions, with a number of them related to health care. Like adverse events, grievances must be evaluated both individually and in aggregate. They provide clues to unsafe systems and providers, even acting as an early warning system regarding safety issues (Paterson, 2013; Pichert, Hickson, & Moore, 2008).

Promptly dealing with individual inmate grievances can often avert future legal action. Even if unfounded, inmate legal claims can tie up considerable time and financial resources establishing and accounting for the actual care provided. Reviewing aggregate reports of

"As a former health care administrator and now as the leader of a risk management consulting firm, I've come to really appreciate the opportunity to spotlight mistakes; certainly not because of the harm or potential for harm, but for the potential they have for preventing harm. It's a wise manager that likes to receive complaints. Just like negative feedback helps all types of organizations identify and improve products and services, paying close attention to the negative experiences in one patient's care can dramatically improve processes and outcomes for many patients to come. If we can move away from blaming and shaming practitioners for errors, and instead reward them for self-reporting in hopes of preventing future harm, we can use what we learn to change processes, redesign the environments of care, create safeguards, and work smarter. That means a higher quality care, fewer adverse events, and better outcomes. Never waste a good mistake!"

— **Michelle Foster Earle, LNFA, ARM, President, OmniSure Consulting Group, Austin, TX** inmate grievances over time can identify latent system issues for proactive attention. For example, accumulating grievances about lack of attention to dental issues may reveal a delay in the sick call request triaging system or a need for more dental staff hours to accommodate the number of requests.

Some correctional settings have a culture that trivializes inmate complaints and ascribes manipulative motivations to all inmates filing grievances. On an individual case basis, this is demeaning; but on an organizational level, disregarding patient complaints in the form of grievances can result in a lost opportunity to reduce error and increase patient safety. Using inmate grievances as an opportunity for system and process improvement supports a patient-centered approach to health care provision and harm reduction. Inmate grievances about health care flow into the risk manage-ment program through the quality improvement program; well-founded grievances provide valuable feedback on many aspects of the clinical program (NCCHC, 2014).

Credentialing and Competency (Scope of Practice)

Competent and appropriately credentialed care providers are the backbone of a safe health care delivery system. An essential element of risk management programs is the confirmation of credentials at the start of employment, followed by an initial evaluation of competence, and an ongoing program to develop competencies of all staff in the organization. It is not uncommon for incompetent providers to seek employment in the correctional system on the mistaken belief that standards are lower when dealing with inmate patients than the general public. Safeguards must be in place to prevent these individuals from entering the correctional health care field.

Credentialing. Credentialing to evaluate the licensure and certification status of a potential staff member should be accomplished prior to hire (Hoffman, 2009). Licensing acts as a safety net for the consumer. Because it is government-regulated, it is a legal requirement for many health care positions. Systems must be in place to assure that practitioners have a free and unencumbered license to practice in the position and in the geographic location of the facility (usually the state). Professional boundaries of licensure differ among states but not among health care settings within jurisdictions; therefore, a physician unable to practice in a traditional setting would also be unqualified to practice in a correctional setting. Indeed, accreditation standards require that "the credential verification process includes inquiry regarding sanctions or disciplinary actions of state boards, employers, and the National Practitioner Data Bank (NPDB)" (NCCHC, 2014, p.39).

Variability of licensure boundaries is most apparent for the LPN/LVN licensure. The types of responsibilities and functions allowable for practical nurses can be wildly different from one state to the next. This is an area of great concern in the correctional setting where limited budgets and oversight can lead to risky practices. As such, careful review of state practice acts for all licensed staff is warranted.

Initial competency. Employers have a responsibility to ensure that new staff members are competent to practice; therefore, employee orientation practices are a part of risk reduction efforts. An organized on-boarding process addressing the knowledge, skill, and attitude necessary for successful job performance ensures consistency and increases safety in care delivery. The orientation program should incorporate major risk concerns in correctional health care as well as those particular to the facility or program. For example, personal safety is a significant concern in the correctional setting. New employees must understand how to activate the facility safety mechanisms and how to be mindful about personal safety.

Ongoing competency. The changing nature of correctional health care requires a process for ongoing competency development and evaluation, including peer review. This can be challenging in a small setting, where there may be only one physician or nurse providing care. In this situation, an outside peer review process is necessary. County jails may be able to partner with the state prison system to accomplish a pool of peer-professionals to review clinical situations and documentation to determine competency. Ongoing competence development is needed when any clinical system is changed. Staff members must understand the reason for the change, the components of the new process, and their role in accomplishing the determined outcome.

Regulatory and Accreditation Compliance

Compliance with regulatory and accreditation standards is another major component of risk management programs. These requirements reflect the standard of practice in the field and provide the structure for delivery of safe patient care.

Regulatory compliance. Government regulatory agencies seek to protect the public from harm through legal requirements and oversight. Correctional health care providers are no different; they must comply with federal, and possibly state, regulations – and the list can be daunting. The following are a few prime examples of agencies and legal acts that must be considered:

- Occupational Safety and Health Administration (OSHA) – use of sharp safety devices; employee injury; environmental chemicals (MSDS)

- Clinical Laboratory Improvement Amendments (CLIA) – onsite laboratory testing

- Patient Self Determination Act (PSA) - consent and advanced directives

- Child Protective Service (CPS) – reporting of abuse or neglect

Accreditation compliance. Although not all correctional health care settings are accredited, accreditation principles are often used as the reference for agency policy and procedure. Accreditation standards are considered standards of practice from a legal perspective. Prudent management of risk ensures that health care delivery in correctional facilities matches accreditation standards as closely as possible. Both the American Correctional Association (ACA, 2010) and the National Commission on Correctional Health Care (NCCHC, 2014) have established accreditation standards for the correctional setting.

Managing Claims: Professional Liability and Civil Rights

Claims management is a significant part of the risk management program. Once a patient makes a claim of injury, the health care entity initiates steps to reduce liability and provide appropriate defense of actions (Barton, 2009). There are significant financial, professional and personal implications to the resolution of these claims. Correctional health care claims can take two forms: professional liability claims and civil rights claims.

Professional Liability Claims. Professional liability claims are the most common claim in traditional health care settings and involve an allegation of professional negligence in an action or omission by a care provider (Hoffman, 2009). To prevail in the case, the claimant (plaintiff) must prove four basic elements:

1. The defendant had a duty to the claimant in their professional capacity;

2. There was a breach of duty in the incident under consideration;

3. This breach of duty caused the injury in question; and

4. The plaintiff suffered damages due to the breach of duty. Damages could include pain, suffering, medical expenses or other losses (Hoffman, 2009).

Duty to a patient is often encapsulated as standard of care. In correctional health care, standard of care is determined by community or constitutional standard. Accreditation standards such as NCCHC or ACA Correctional Health Care Standards are often considered the standard of care in correctional health care litigation. Expert testimony is then used to determine the standard of care for a particular professional in a clinical situation.

Civil Rights Claims. Civil rights claims are more common in the correctional health care setting as these claim abrogation of the plaintiff's constitutional rights under the Eighth or Fourteenth Amendment to the United States Constitution. Civil rights claims are adjudicated through Section 1983 of the Civil Rights Act of 1871, which provides for civil liability on any person who deprives another citizen of their constitutional rights (Moore, 2013). The Eighth Amendment to the US Constitution protects citizens from cruel and unusual criminal punishment. In the landmark ruling regarding *Estelle v. Gamble* in 1976, the Supreme Court determined that withholding necessary medical care constituted cruel and unusual punishment as defined by this amendment. Case law following *Estelle* established three basic rights to sentenced inmates:

1. the right to access care;

2. the right to receive the care that was ordered; and

3. the right to a professional health care judgment (Rold, 2007).

In addition, *Estelle* prompted the Court to establish the term "deliberate indifference to serious medical need." Deliberate indifference requires the defendant to both know about and disregard a serious health need. A serious medical need is defined as one that is diagnosed as needing treatment and/or a condition so obvious as to be recognized by even a lay person as needing medical care (Rold, 2007). Another definition some find useful is: A serious medical need is a valid health condition that, without timely medical intervention, will cause (1) unnecessary pain, (2) measurable deterioration in function (including organ function), (3) death, or (4) substantial risk to the public health (Greifinger, 2006).

As the Eighth Amendment is applicable only to sentenced citizens, the health care rights of pre-trial jail detainees were established under the Fourteenth Amendment's due process clause. In *Bell v. Wolfish* in 1979, the Court established that persons confined in a jail must be provided with reasonably safe conditions of confinement. A later ruling, Farmer v. Brennan in 1994, clearly stated that medical care was a part of the required safe conditions. Therefore, withholding necessary medical care to a detainee was determined to be a form of punishment imposed before the citizen was convicted of any crime (Farber, 2007). Although covered under different Amendments, the constitutional right to adequate health care is now equally established for both sentenced and pre-trial prisoners.

A civil claim of deliberate indifference is more difficult to prove than a claim of professional negligence because it typically requires a determination of conscious disregard; however, inmates frequently resort to this type of claim for several reasons. Section 1983 claims have a longer shelf life, as medical malpractice claims are governed by state law and can have a shorter timeframe for filing. In addition, plaintiff attorneys like Section 1983 cases because their reasonable fees, if they prevail, must be covered by the defendant independent of the amount of the award to the plaintiff, as opposed to a proportional contingency. This element of the law allows for the pursuit of "smaller" claims that might not otherwise be considered (Loevy, 2004).

Prison Litigation Reform Act (PLRA). The number of lawsuits filed by inmates greatly increased from 1970 to 1995, when more than 40,000 inmate claims clogged the legal system (Taylor, 2000) and inspired reform efforts. The PLRA of 1995 aimed to reduce frivolous and unnecessary inmate lawsuits by creating some boundaries on the types and frequency of legal claims.

There are several important points about PLRA in relation to risk management. In particular, the Act requires that an inmate first use the internal grievance system to the full extent (including any appeals process) before taking legal action on a claim. It is important for a correctional facility to have a clear written internal grievance policy and procedure known to all staff and inmates - and to consistently follow it. If an inmate plaintiff has not exhausted internal grievance processes prior to making a claim, it will likely be thrown out upon review. The PLRA allows a case to be screened by the court and dismissed as frivolous even before the defense is required to reply (Boston, 2012).

Upfront filing fees are generally waived or greatly decreased for inmates due to poverty. This clause also encourages inmates to file civil rights claims rather than professional liability claims. However, after an inmate has three lawsuits dismissed as "frivolous, malicious, or failing to state a claim for relief", this waiver is exhausted. Further filings will require the full fee to be paid upfront (Boston, 2012).

Claims Process

The claims process has similar steps, no matter the type of legal claim (Barton, 2009).

Initiation of the claim. Written notice of a legal claim can arrive at any time and to any member of the organization. Everyone in the system should be aware of the process for handling legal claims, including contact person(s) and how rapidly to act. It is helpful to have a written guideline or policy and procedure to work from. The health services manager and medical director should meet with risk management to review the claims management process for a specific case.

Claim investigation. Once a claim is reported, investigation of the alleged injury begins. An internal team, led by risk management, performs the investigation - consisting of medical record review, interviews with staff involved in the situation, and possibly outside expert review of the case. In the correctional setting, internal claim investigation may also involve custody documentation, officer interview, and video and audio recording review. For example, the patient might claim a mobility injury but be seen on camera playing basketball with other inmates in the yard.

Liability determination. Once a full investigation has been completed, an internal determination of liability is made. This may involve a claims committee or review of the investigation materials by legal counsel.

Settlement or litigation. Liability determination is a key component in deciding to settle a case or move to litigation. At any time during this process, the defense team may choose to submit a motion for summary judgment that asks the judge to dismiss all or part of the claim without trial due to a lack of substantive evidence.

Summary

Correctional health care is fraught with legal risk. The structure of correctional health care is built on a foundation of legal and legislative precedent, resulting in a defensive posture in determining appropriate care. The patient safety movement, developed in traditional practice settings over the last two decades, provides a more robust and fruitful organizational framework for managing risk in correctional health care. By focusing on the patient, efforts to reduce harm lead to decreased clinical error and therefore reduced litigation risk. Likewise, a patient safety focus will naturally lead to the improved clinical processes and outcomes desired by continuous quality improvement programs. Therefore, a patient safety management model benefits all stakeholders in correctional health care.

References

American Correctional Association (ACA). (2010). *Standards supplement 2010.* Alexandria, VA: American Correctional Association.

Aspden, P. & Institute of Medicine (IOM) Committee on Data Standards for Patient Safety. (2004). *Patient safety achieving a new standard for care.* Washington, DC: National Academies Press.

Barnsteiner, J.H. (2012). Safety. In G. Sherwood (Ed.), *Quality and safety in nursing: A competency approach to improving outcomes* (pp. 149–169). Chichester, West Sussex, UK: Wiley-Blackwell.

Barton, E. (2009). Basic claims management. In R. Carroll (Ed.), *Risk management handbook for health care organizations* (pp. 367–379). San Francisco, CA: Jossey-Bass.

Boston, J. (2012, February 20). *The Prison Litigation Reform Act. The Legal Aid Society.* Retrieved from http://www.illinoislegaladvocate.org/uploads/8032theplra0312.pdf.

Burhans, L.D., Chastain, K., & George, J.L. (2012). Just culture and nursing regulation: Learning to improve patient safety. *Journal of Nursing Regulation, 2*(4), 43–49.

Carroll, J.S. & Rudolph, J.W. (2006). Design of high reliability organizations in health care. *Quality and Safety in Health Care, 15*(suppl_1), i4–i9. doi:10.1136/qshc.2005.015867

Carroll, R. (Ed.). (2009). *Risk management handbook for health care organizations* (Student ed.). San Francisco, CA: Jossey-Bass.

Chassin, M.R. & Becher, E.C. (2002). The wrong patient. *Annals of Internal Medicine, 136*(11), 826–833.

Dekker, S. (2011). *Patient safety: a human factors approach.* Boca Raton, FL: CRC Press.

Department of Veterans Affairs National Center for Patient Safety. (2009, December). *Root cause analysis tools.* Retrieved from http://www.patientsafety.va.gov/CogAids/RCA/index.html - page-1.

ECRI Institute. (2009, July). Risk management, quality improvement, and patient safety. *Healthcare Risk Control, 2*, 1-15. Retrieved from https://www.ecri.org/Documents/secure/Risk_Quality_Patient_Safety.pdf.

Edmondson, A.C. (2004). Learning from failure in health care: Frequent opportunities, pervasive barriers. *Quality and Safety in Health Care, 13*(suppl 2), ii3–ii9. doi:10.1136/qshc.2003.009597

Emanuel, L., Berwick, D., Conway, J., Combes, J., Hatlie, M., Leape, L., … Walton, M. (2008). What exactly is patient safety? *Advances in Patient Safety: New Directions and Alternative Approaches, 1.* Retrieved from http://ahrq.hhs.gov/downloads/pub/advances2/vol1/Advances-Emanuel-Berwick_110.pdf.

Farber, B.J. (2007). Civil liability for inadequate prisoner medical care: An Introduction. *AELE Monthly Law Journal, 2007*(9), 301–311.

Finkelman, A.W. (2009). *Teaching IOM: Implications of the Institute of Medicine Reports for Nursing Education* (2nd ed.). Silver Spring, MD: American Nurses Association.

Greifinger, R.B. (2006). Health care quality through care management. In M. Puisis (Ed.), *Clinical practice in correctional medicine (2nd ed.,* pp. 510-519). St. Louis: Mosby

Greifinger, R.B. (2007). Thirty years since Estelle v. Gamble: Looking forward, not wayward. In R. B. Greifinger (Ed.), *Public health behind bars—From prisons to communities* (pp. 1-10). New York: Springer

Henriksen, K., Dayton, E., Keyes, M. A., Carayon, P., & Hughes, R. (2008). Understanding adverse events: A human factors framework. In R. G. Hughes (Ed.), *Patient safety and quality: An evidence based handbook for nurses.* Rockville, MD: Agency for Healthcare Research and Quality. Retrieved from www.ncbi.nlm.nih.gov/books/NBK2666/

Hoffman, P. (2009). Health care legal concepts. In R. Carroll (Ed.), *Risk management handbook for health care organizations* (Student ed., pp. 115–157). San Francisco, CA: Jossey-Bass.

Institute of Medicine Committee on Quality of Health Care in America. (2000). *To err is human: Building a safer health system.* Washington, D.C.: The National Academies Press.

Institute of Medicine Committee on Quality of Health Care in America. (2001). *Crossing the quality chasm: A new health system for the 21st century.* Washington, D.C.: National Academy Press. Retrieved from http://search. ebscohost.com/login.aspx?direct=true&scope=site&db=nlebk&db=nlabk&AN =86916.

Loevy, J. (2004). Section 1983 Litigation in a nutshell: Make a case out of it! *The Journal of the DuPage County Bar Association, 17.* Retrieved from www.dcbabrief.org/vol171004art2.html.

McCaffrey, J. & Hagg-Rickert, S. (2009). Development of a risk management program. In R. Carroll (Ed.), *Risk management handbook for health care organizations* (Student ed., pp. 1–30). San Francisco, CA: Jossey-Bass.

Moen, R. D., & Norman, C. L. (2011). Circling back. *Quality Control and Applied Statistics, 56*(3), 265–266.

Moore, J. (2013). Legal considerations in correctional nursing. In L. Schoenly & C.M. Knox (Eds.), *Essentials of correctional nursing* (pp. 39–55). New York, NY: Springer.

Murphy, D., Shannon, K., & Pugliese, G. (2009). Patient safety and the risk management professional: New challenges and opportunities. In R. Carroll (Ed.), *Risk management handbook for health care organizations* (Student ed., pp. 87–113). San Francisco, CA: Jossey-Bass.

Napier, J. & Youngberg, B. (2011). Risk management and patient safety: The synergy and the tension. In B. Youngberg (Ed.), *Principles of risk management and patient safety* (pp. 3–11). Boston, MA: Jones and Bartlett Learning.

National Commission on Correctional Health Care (NCCHC). (2014). *Standards for health services in prisons, 2014.* Chicago, IL: National Commission on Correctional Health Care.

Paterson, R. (2013). Not so random: Patient complaints and "frequent flier" doctors. *BMJ Quality & Safety, 22*(7), 525–527. doi:10.1136/bmjqs-2013-001902

Pichert, J.W., Hickson, G., & Moore, I. (2008). Using patient complaints to promote patient safety. In K. Henriksen, J.B. Battles, M.A. Keyes, & M.L. Grady (Eds.), *Advances in patient safety: New directions and alternative approaches (Vol. 2: Culture and redesign).* Rockville, MD: Agency for Healthcare Research and Quality. Retrieved from http://www.ncbi.nlm.nih.gov/books/ NBK43703/

Reason, J. (2000). Human error: models and management. *BMJ: British Medical Journal, 320*(7237), 768.

Reed, K. & May, R. (2011, March). *HealthGrades Patient Safety in American Hospitals Study.* Retrieved from www.visimobile.com/wp-content/uploads/2012/05/Patient-Safety-In-American-Hospitals-Study-2011-Healthgrades_201203051.pdf

Rold, W.J. (2007). Thirty years after *Estelle v. Gamble*: A legal retrospective. *Journal of Correctional Health Care, 14*(1), 11–20. doi:10.1177/1078345807309616

Rothstein, M.A. (2010). Currents in contemporary bioethics. *The Journal of Law, Medicine & Ethics, 38*(4), 871–874. doi:10.1111/j.1748-720X.2010.00540.x

Sparnon, E. & Marella, W.M. (2012). The role of the electronic health record in patient safety events. *Pennsylvania Patient Safety Advisor, 9*(4), 113–121.

Spath, P. (2011). *Error reduction in health care: A systems approach to improving patient safety.* San Francisco, CA: Jossey-Bass.

Stern, M.F., Greifinger, R.B., & Mellow, J. (2010). Patient safety: Moving the bar in prison health care standards. *American Journal of Public Health, 100*(11), 2103.

Taylor, K. (2000). Prison Litigation Reform Act's administrative exhaustion requirement: Closing the money damages loophole. *Washington University Law Review, 78*, 955-78.

The Joint Commission. (2012, June 27). *Joint Commission Center for Transforming Healthcare releases tool to tackle miscommunication among caregivers.* Retrieved from www.jointcommission.org/ center_transforming_healthcare_tst_hoc/

Thompson, J.H. (2010). Today's deliberate indifference: Providing attention without providing treatment to prisoners with serious medical needs. Harvard Civil Rights-Civil Liberties Law Review, 45, 635.

Wachter, R.M. (2012). *Understanding patient safety* (2nd ed.). New York, NY: Mcgraw-Hill.

2 Environment of Care

The environment of care is of particular concern in a correctional setting. Unlike traditional health care, most correctional care delivery takes place in an environment managed by others. Correctional professionals have a world view nurtured by their values and beliefs, which can compete or conflict with the role of health care and lead to patient safety challenges. Organizational culture must support mutual goals of health care and custody so that the environment promotes safety. This environment, then, supports the other domains of patient safety (Figure 2.1). The basic principle underlying the environment of care domain of patient safety is promoting a Just Culture in a learning organization (Table 2.1). Building this Just Culture involves gaining an understanding of an organization's prevailing culture and incorporating concepts from a culture of respect and a patient safety culture. These cultural components provide a foundation for development of a Just Culture.

Figure 2.1 A Patient Safety Model of Health Care

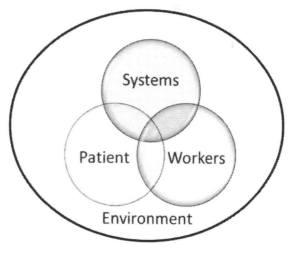

Adapted from Emanuel et al., 2008

Organizational Culture

Culture is described as the commonly-held attitudes and practices of a group (Spath, 2011). An organization's culture establishes norms of behavior that are approved, allowed, or ignored. It also establishes behaviors that are punished or rewarded. This culture is absorbed by staff members and affects their attitudes and actions. It is often invisible to the eye, yet pervades the environment as the aroma of an individual's perfume might fill an elevator. Everyone is affected by it, but no one sees nor mentions it. If an organization's 'scent' negatively affects teamwork, collaboration, and communication, it can be difficult to remove. The removal effort is worthwhile, however, as patient safety is improved when an organization's culture supports open, transparent commun-ication and mutual goals.

Table 2.1. Domains and Principles of Patient Safety

Domain of Patient Safety	Principle of Patient Safety
Environment of Care	A Just Culture in a Learning Organization
Systems for Therapeutic Action	High Reliability System Design Communication and Teamwork
Recipient of Care	Patient-Centered Care
Health Care Workers	Competent Care Providers Communication and Teamwork

The diverse perspectives of health care professionals often complicate organizational culture change. Physicians and nurses have professional viewpoints about their roles – and the roles of others in the organization – that are often aligned but can sometimes be at odds in a particular care situation. In correctional health care, the security perspective overlaying the care environment also affects organizational culture. It may be difficult to move toward open and honest communication of error in a command-and-control environment. Health care is most often accomplished through collaboration and a team approach. But, if health care staff arrive in a housing unit to medically manage a situation, custody staff may not expect to dialog about possible cause and intervention options; that is, however, a cultural norm for most who work in health care.

Communication can be further hampered if health team leadership also has a dictatorial demeanor. Team members in a subordinate position may respond by being indirect in expressing recommendations, thus compromising clarity. In fact, nurses tend to favor compromise in a conflict situation, while unlicensed staff favor conflict avoidance (Sportsman & Hamilton, 2007). Although these styles can be helpful in some situations, compromising or avoiding conflict over patient safety issues can lead to clinical error. If custody staff are discouraged from speaking up about concerns of ethical or safe treatment within the facility, it will be even more difficult for health care staff to address these issues openly.

The correctional organizational structure adds an additional cultural component to safe health care delivery. Relationship-building is important to develop a full understanding of each discipline's perspective in care provision. This includes valuing each discipline's expertise, professional ethics, and goals. Mutual respect and open communication among correctional and health care professionals are important cultural elements of an effective organization. The unity of diverse perspectives works best when all participants know their role and 'play their position' on the team.

Gender, ethnic background, and generational differences contribute to organizational culture. The diversity of perspectives among various cultures and generations can affect underlying assumptions and responses to situations (Clochesy, 2008). Tension among genders can also affect culture. Corrections is still a male-dominated profession, and some settings continue to struggle with acceptance of women in leadership positions (Nicholas, 2013). These differences have to be taken into consideration as part of the efforts to move toward a patient safety organizational culture.

Culture of Respect

Respect is foundational to a healthy organizational culture. Incivility in the workplace is a threat to the smooth operation of any organization. Coworker rudeness can decrease concentration, reduce communication, and inhibit collaboration (Flin, 2010; Painter, 2013). Intimidating and disruptive behaviors by fellow staff members hinder the open working relationship necessary in a high-performance industry with pressures from required cost containment, embedded hierarchies, and threatened or realized litigation (Alert, 2008). Efforts at developing a patient safety and Just Culture must also address the interpersonal relationships of the individuals within the system.

Hostility among coworkers provides an additional threat to patient safety. A connection between workplace hostility

> "Good patient care is good custody. In a correctional environment one does not exist without the other."
> – Art Beeler, Former Warden, Federal Medical Center, Butner, North Carolina

and clinical error has long been identified (Alert, 2008; Grissinger, 2011). As such, the American Medical Association (AMA) has charged the medical profession with taking leadership in reducing workplace hostility in health care. It outlines appropriate and inappropriate behaviors in a Model Medical Staff Code of

Conduct that is applicable to the correctional setting (AMA, 2008). A code of conduct makes clear the organizational expectations for healthy workplace communication and describes steps that can be taken when abusive, coercive or harassing communication is experienced. The Joint Commission now requires that a hospital implement such a code of conduct and take steps to manage inappropriate and disruptive behaviors of all staff (Alert, 2008).

Interdisciplinary collaborative relationships must be nurtured to survive the many stresses of health care delivery. The American Organization of Nurse Executives (AONE; 2005) suggests nine guiding principles that encourage, in particular, nurse-physician collaborative relationships (Table 2.2). These principles, however, are applicable for all health care staff, including pharmacists, therapists and support staff. In fact, they have application in custody-health care interactions as well.

In the correctional setting, workplace hostility can be pervasive throughout the facility – among custody and health care staff alike. Hostility between custody and health care may accompany a definite "us

Table 2.2 AONE Guiding Principles

1. Interdisciplinary collaborative relationships are promoted, nurtured and sustained.

2. Excellence in relationship-building begins with hiring, continues with learning and developing together and is reinforced over time.

3. This requires that practitioners be proficient in communication skills, leadership skills, problem solving, conflict management, utilizing their emotional intelligence and functioning within a team culture.

4. The organization has a specific system for reward, recognition and celebration.

5. The organization supports the "Platinum Rule"* with a specific Professional Code of Conduct that includes a system to support it. A No-Tolerance standard exists for those unable to adhere to the Code.

6. The organization creates and supports a "Just & Fair" environment.

7. The work of all professional caregivers is seen as interdependent and collegial.

8. Cross-discipline job discovery is supported and encouraged.

9. Patient-focused care and better patient outcomes are the organizing force behind creating a collaborative environment.

*treat others as they want to be treated
From American Organization of Nurse Executives, 2005 , pg.1

vs. them" mentality. Bullying of the powerless, be it the inmate population or support staff, may be the predominant working culture; yet communication and collaboration among all disciplines is necessary for adequate patient safety. Even well-meaning health care staff can be drawn to respond in kind to intimidating behavior, be it from the patient, custody staff, or health care peers. Staff may need education and coaching to develop skills to appropriately respond to intimidating behaviors in the work setting.

Health care staff may also need specific guidance in how to respond to uncivil or demeaning behavior viewed during the course of delivering care. Team members who have less powerful positions in the organizational structure may, nonetheless, need to act on what they have witnessed. For example, if an LPN views an inappropriate use of force by custody officers, what actions can be taken? Discussing the potential for these experiences and the appropriate actions that need to be taken early in this nurse's tenure can benefit both the nurse and her patient in this situation.

Interventions that encourage a culture of respect in a traditional health care setting can also be applied to the larger correctional organization by the combined efforts and role modeling of both custody and health care leadership in the institution. Key characteristics of a successful code of conduct include emphasis on fairness, consistency, graded response to infraction, a specific restorative process, and a surveillance mechanism (Leape et al., 2012). In that regard, health care ethical codes will have principles in common with correctional officer codes such as the ACA Code of Ethics which begins by stating that "the American Correctional Association expects of its members unfailing honesty, respect for the dignity and individuality of human beings, and a commitment to professional and compassionate service" (ACA, 1994, pg. 1).

Patient Safety Culture

A patient safety culture builds on a culture of respect and is non-punitive in nature; valuing accountability, honesty, and mutual respect (Barnsteiner, 2012). In fact, one author described a safety culture as one that "allows the boss to hear bad news" (Dekker, 2011, p. 100). Many factors must be active for the "bad news" to reach the boss. First, a communication system must be in place throughout all levels of the organization. Then, a commitment to patient safety must extend through these levels, enabling difficult-to-hear information to be shared. This requires open communication based on trust and positive regard.

Organizational culture can be categorized into three types (Table 2.3). These types can provide a description of the cultural components that affect patient safety. A generative culture encourages the open flow of information, while bureaucratic and pathological cultures thwart these efforts, striving instead to discourage change or cover up failures. Determining organizational culture type can assist in determining priorities when working to improve patient safety.

1. Wachter (2012) described four key elements of a safety culture:

2. Acknowledgement of the high-risk, error-prone nature of an organization's activities;

3. A blame-free environment where individuals are able to report errors or near-miss events without fear of reprimand or punishment;

4. An expectation of collaboration across ranks to seek solutions to vulnerabilities;

5. A willingness on the part of the organization to direct resources to addressing safety concerns.

Table 2.3 Safety Characteristics of Organizational Cultures Types

Culture Type	Characteristics
Generative	Encourages upward flow of information; Rewards the messengers; Focuses on collective mindfulness of work hazards; Expects bad things to happen and prepares for them; Best for patient safety outcomes.
Bureaucratic	Operates "by the book" and dislikes new ideas and approaches; Does not kill the messenger but considers bad news a problem; Relies on administrative controls to remain safe; Majority of organizations.
Pathological	Shirks safety responsibilities; Does not really want to know about problems; Kills the messenger and marginalizes whistleblowers; Punishes or covers up failures; Most unsafe of cultures.

Adapted from Reason, 2008

Some correctional cultures may expect perfect work, even though the human condition is fraught with error. Acknowledging the high-risk nature of health care, along with the human tendency toward imperfection, should lead to organizational activities that look for root cause and seek out system design improvements to reduce error. An expectation of perfect work leads to dismissal of individuals involved in a clinical error, therefore allowing system issues to go unattended and resulting in continuing troubles. Correctional accrediting bodies understand this vulnerability in the correctional health care setting and encourage the creation of a culture of patient safety in accrediting standards (NCCHC, 2014).

Requiring unrealistically perfect work also leads to a blaming environment intent on seeking out and dismissing "bad apple" employees. This culture then initiates fear of reprisal and a resultant silence in the face of error identification. Individuals fear reprimand, punishment, and termination if errors are identified.

As discussed earlier, open collaboration among the various levels of the organization is a key component to a patient safety culture. Staff must feel free to speak openly about potentially unsafe situations and initiate dialog leading to improvements rather than work-arounds or other responses to unsafe situations.

It is critical for leadership to understand patient safety principles and be willing to support system-change efforts for lasting improvement. If only staff and front-line members of the organization see the benefit of patient safety efforts, they are likely to be unsupported at higher levels, thus resulting in reversion to prior processes over time. Both management and staff must collectively understand, support, and implement these strategies – with full support from all parties – to have an effective patient safety program. Basic changes to practice must have organizational support to survive. Thus, if health care leadership is convinced that pre-pouring medications is an unsafe practice, security leadership must be willing to consider longer nurse activity in the housing units for direct delivery of medications from a mobile unit.

Just Culture

The movement to a patient safety culture, with open communication of error and blame-free environment, leads to concerns about errors that, indeed, result from willful disregard of safety mechanisms. Reckless behavior on the part of health care practitioners needs to be corrected in order to improve patient safety. The addition of professional accountability to the patient safety culture framework created the concept of Just Culture. A Just Culture strikes a balance between a no-blame culture that does not hold individuals accountable for their actions and the traditional, overly-punitive "bad apple" culture that seeks to ascribe blame for error to individual practitioners (Morris, 2011). A Just Culture evaluates practitioner involvement as part of a balanced investigation of events, acknowledging that at the sharp end of a clinical error may be unhealthy normative staff behaviors such as shortcuts or reckless behaviors such as blatant disregard for standard safety rules (Wachter, 2012). These situations must be dealt with along with the systems that perpetuate clinical error.

A Just Culture in health care was first advocated by Marx (2001) in a classic work that identified types of individual behaviors that might result in clinical error. Understanding the four behavioral concepts can help in the determination of the root cause of a clinical error under evaluation (Table 2.4). Licensure boards have used this continuum to evaluate clinician behaviors that could result in disciplinary action (Burhans, Chastain, & George, 2012).

Table 2.4 Behavioral Concepts Involved in Clinical Error

Behavioral Concept	Description
Human Error	Someone did other than what they should have done; Does not ascribe intentionality; Mistakes, lapses, slips.
Negligent Conduct	Indicates that the individual should have been aware of the risk and consequence of the action and, therefore, is culpable for the outcome of the error; A failure to recognize unjustified risk.
Reckless Conduct	A conscious disregard for a significant risk of error - this is a higher degree than negligent conduct, where the individual should have known the risk.
Intentional Rule Violation	Knowing violation of safety rules for performing a task.

Adapted from Marx, 2001

Caring for the Second Victim

A Just Culture not only considers human accountability in clinical errors but also attends to the individual aftermath of involvement in the error. A culture that seeks to be transparent in dealing with inevitable human error will be sensitive to the post-traumatic aftermath of involvement in patient harm. Health care workers directly involved in the error are often a second victim in the error episode, suffering extreme stress, depression, anxiety and other psychological effects. They are likely to punish themselves for the failure and relive the incident repeatedly. Compounding this personal punishment, other health care professionals may distance themselves from this second victim, withdrawing support when it is most needed (Dekker, 2012).

To overcome the aftermath of error, clinicians must be able to trust that the organization will treat them fairly, with compassion and understanding. This includes respectful, supportive care during the evaluation and resolution of the episode (Denham, 2007). In a Just Culture, organizational transparency provides an opportunity for the individual at the sharp end of the incident to contribute to the changes that would lead to future error prevention (Denham, 2007).

A study of various professional health care staff involved in a clinical error at Johns Hopkins Medical Center revealed desired organizational support strategies deemed most helpful in obtaining personal resolution of the incident (Edrees, Paine, Feroli, & Wu, 2011). The most frequently indicated actions were prompt debriefing with crisis intervention, opportunity to discuss any ethical concerns about the event, input into system changes, timely information about the upcoming evaluation processes, and access to psychological and emotional support (Table 2.5).

Table 2.5 Organizational Support Strategies for Staff Involved in a Clinical Error

Strategy	Percent Agreement
Prompt debriefing following the event	74.5
Opportunity to discuss ethical concerns about the event	45.7
Safe opportunity to contribute insights into preventing similar events	44.7
Clear and timely information about the follow-up processes	43.6
Access to psychological/psychiatric services	35.1
Formal emotional support	35.1

Adapted from Edrees et al., 2011

Reaching an Optimum Environment of Care

Evaluating Culture

A frequent starting point for implementing a patient safety culture is to evaluate the current organizational culture. This evaluation can lead to a prioritized list of necessary changes and set a path toward appropriate culture change. In addition, a culture evaluation can elevate awareness of safety concern for front-line staff (Nieva

& Sorra, 2003). Several culture evaluation tools are available; however, most lack adequate validation for use in a correctional health care setting (Pronovost & Sexton, 2005). Extensive testing of two tools – the Safety Attitudes Questionnaire and the AHRQ Survey of Patient Safety – suggests they may be helpful for patient safety culture evaluation in the correctional setting.

The Safety Attitude Questionnaire (SAQ) developed by the University of Texas assesses caregiver attitudes along six factors of patient safety: Teamwork Climate, Safety Climate, Perception of Management, Job Satisfaction, Working Conditions, and Stress Recognition (Sexton et al., 2006). Participants record their attitudes toward 60 items using a five-point likert-like scale. A shorter ambulatory care version is available with 19 items. In a review of nine available patient safety culture evaluation tools, only the SAQ had published data linking climate scores to positive patient outcomes (Colla, 2005). The extensive evaluation of this tool makes it a good survey option in the correctional setting. The SAQ is also a credible tool for use in serial climate evaluations and as an outcome tool when implementing climate change projects (Watts, Percarpio, West, & Mills, 2010).

Another safety culture evaluation tool that may be helpful for the correctional setting is the AHRQ Survey of Patient Safety (SOPS). This tool surveys staff perception of 12 dimensions of the patient safety culture. Although developed for the traditional hospital setting, use in long-term care is also reported (Wagner, Capezuti, & Rice, 2009). A comparative database through AHRQ allows benchmarking among institutions.

Finally, consider use of a corrections-specific organizational assessment program such as the APEX Assessment Tools for Organizational Assessment (Bogue & Cebula, 2012). Although not specific to patient safety, these tools are widely accepted within the corrections profession and can gain custody leadership support should there be apprehension about the project. Values inherent in the Organizational Culture Assessment Instrument, a part of the APEX evaluation process, are compatible with those of a patient safety culture.

Issues of Survey Administration

Care is needed in planning and implementing a patient culture assessment. If this is a first effort toward improving culture, this needs to be a positive experience. Formal and informal leaders and all stakeholders should be involved in the process and have a full understanding of the need for, and uses of, survey results (Nieva & Sorra, 2003). This will encourage participation. In order to obtain an accurate representation of the safety culture, a response rate of at least 60% is recommended (Pronovost & Sexton, 2005). A response rate of less than 60% may result in documentation of opinion and not organizational culture.

Attention to the procedure for data collection will also assist in obtaining a valid and reliable result. Both full-time and part-time managers and staff should be a part of the survey. Survey responses should be anonymous and uncoerced. Staff should be given time to complete the survey away from patient care duties and not be prepared to provide "correct" answers through any pre-assessment educational programing (Nieva & Sorra, 2003).

Front-line staff need to hear the results of the survey. This communication can encourage participation in future surveys and assist in garnering enthusiasm for organizational change activities. Sustained culture change is difficult at best, requiring the continued involvement of leadership and stakeholders. To improve impact, feedback can be combined with action planning in multi-disciplinary focus groups (Nieva & Sorra, 2003).

"Executive/Management Walkrounds are essential to changing and creating a Just Culture. Leadership visibility lets staff know that management is present, engaged and interested in the daily routine tasks and challenges of providing correctional health care in their facility. The "Walkround" is not necessarily the time to solve everyone's perceived problems at that exact moment; however, it is a time to gather information about problems as well as acknowledge the workload and other challenges. "Walking around" allows leadership to be aware of and better understand the present and ongoing issues, which is the first step to solving problems, turning around the culture, and ultimately improving patient safety."

– **Kim Pearson, RN, MHA, MBA, CCHP, Orange County, California**

Safety Culture Best Practices

Once a baseline culture assessment has been conducted, thoughts turn toward options for activities to improve the organization's patient safety culture. Several best practices for the traditional hospital setting show promise for use in correctional health care. Use of these tools has been found to improve communication about safety hazards, transparency, teamwork, and leadership (Weaver et al., 2013). Because these interventions are often implemented as a bundle, the specific result of the action is difficult to determine; however, evidence from a review of 33 studies supports effectiveness of the following interventions for improving patient safety culture. "The best evidence to date seems to include strategies comprising multiple components that incorporate team training and mechanisms to support team communication and include executive engagement in front-line safety walkrounds" (Weaver et al., 2013, p. 373).

Correctional health care experts confirm the need for addressing organizational culture to improve patient safety. Proposed patient safety standards for the correctional setting include establishing patient safety as a governing principle in written policy and actively involving clinical leadership in identifying and resolving patient safety issues (Stern, Greifinger, & Mellow, 2010). NCCHC accrediting standards also provide support for culture change to improve patient safety. Discussion of Patient Safety Standard B-02 emphasizes the role of organizational leadership in communicating a culture of patient safety to line staff (NCCHC, 2014).

Team training. Team training consists of multi-disciplinary group skill development in communication and teamwork. This training can involve classroom and self-education processes but is most effective when combined with simulation (Cumin, Boyd, Webster, & Weller, 2013; Fagan, 2012). A simulation team learning experience can be as simple as a mock code or disaster drill. An important element of team training using simulation is to emphasize the need for communication and teamwork in the vignette and debriefing process. Team training can reveal difficulties in team dynamics that affect the safety culture. The interpersonal relationships, as well as the communication activities, are an important part of the assessment process.

Executive walkrounds. Executive or interdisciplinary walkrounds that focus on patient safety issues have been found to improve organizational culture (Frankel et al., 2003). Leadership visibility can improve staff morale and leadership influence; both important for culture change. Leadership visibility establishes commitment to patient safety when walkrounds are focused specifically on engaging staff in the environment of care on patient safety issues and concerns. In addition, executive walkrounds demonstrate a leadership Just Culture and transparency – both necessary components of a patient safety climate (Thomas, Sexton, Neilands, Frankel, & Helmreich, 2005).

Unit-based programs. Evidence is growing that a unit-based approach to improving patient safety culture is effective. A systematic review of patient safety literature found evidence of sustained improvements in infection and mortality rates after implementation of the Comprehensive Unit-based Safety Program (CUSP) advocated by AHRQ (Weaver et al., 2013). It can be said that all culture is local. The CUSP model focuses on smaller organizational units, such as multi-disciplinary work teams, to develop skills in implementing evidence-based patient safety practices. This program has seen success in many traditional health care settings and may apply to the correctional setting (Agency for Healthcare Research and Quality, 2012).

The Physical Environment of Care

Although most concern for the care environment in patient safety hinges on organizational culture, the physical environment must also be considered in corrections. Many correctional facilities were not designed with health care delivery in mind, and obstacles to patient safety are pervasive. For example, a primary concern in the care delivery in a secure environment is staff safety. In fact, health care team members are restricted from delivering emergency care until the surrounding area is evaluated for personal danger. This can be morally stressful for professionals trained to focus solely on the needs of the patient.

In addition to personal safety issues, the physical environment may make it difficult to perform normal patient safety checks, such as having a second staff member available to check the dosage of a dangerous medication prior to administration or being able to monitor a patient after the delivery of a first medication dose.

The restrictive nature of a secure environment may require health care staff to rely on housing officers to detect patient changes that indicate a need for medical attention. In many smaller facilities, staff members must manage urgent situations autonomously with telephone access to advanced practice professionals. Security barriers may reduce patient visibility in sub-acute settings such as infirmary or holding areas. There may be limited access to hand washing stations. The inconvenience of extra steps and effort to uphold standard patient safety principles in a geographically challenging layout can lead to hazardous work-arounds or a culture of low expectation among care providers.

A Learning Organization

Senge (1990) originally conceptualized a learning organization as one that encouraged systems thinking, team learning, personal mastery, a shared vision, and mental models to effect positive evolution and change. This learning organization structure can be used to focus on patient safety within health care.

Through leadership from the National Institutes of Corrections, progress is underway in moving correctional organizations toward a learning organization framework (NIC, 2014). Correctional leaders are challenged to include learning organization principles in practice (Christensen, 2004). This professional dialog can be leveraged to provide support for learning organization initiatives within individual facilities.

Patient safety is enhanced when organizations learn from clinical errors. Just like individuals, systems make errors, too; therefore, organizational learning, in addition to individual learning, is needed to prevent future harm (Rivard, Rosen, & Carroll, 2006). Organizational learning is described as a "transformational process that seeks to help organizations develop and use knowledge to change and improve themselves on an ongoing basis" (Claridge, Cook, & Hale, 2008 p. 9). This transformation is necessary to improve the patient safety culture in an organization.

Two orders of learning have been identified in organizations. First-ordered learning takes place at the front line where groups and individuals who are delivering care make changes in their routines. This correlates with the sharp end of care delivery – the intersection of patient and professional. Second-ordered organizational learning involves learning among groups and divisions at the system level (Tucker & Edmondson, 2003). At this level, organizational learning improves organizational routines, or the recognizable patterns of actions involving multiple players (Rivard et al., 2006). Both orders of learning must be present in an organization to effectively reduce patient harm.

Surprisingly, effective error-reduction strategies at the first order of the organization may thwart second-order learning in a health care organization. Tucker & Edmonson (2003) contend that nursing vigilance, unit efficiency concerns, and empowerment can actually work against organizational learning by continually fixing issues at the first order and thus never moving a risky process to the organizational level of concern. Effective first-order learning, then, should also include communication of these efforts to higher levels in the organization.

Both single- and double-loop learning is possible in organizational learning (Figure 2.2). In single-loop learning, changes are made to action strategies and techniques, based on the outcome of a process. In a health care organization, this might involve adapting various adjustments to a new process to help it succeed at the site level without fundamentally changing the process. For example, multi-disciplinary walkrounds may be initiated in the infirmary, with an adjusted schedule that meets the needs of various discipline participation. The team learns to adjust to the new process.

Double-loop learning involves organizational learning encompassing the goals, values and conceptual framework of the organization. This is a deeper change that involves the underlying system within an organization (Hovlid, Bukve, Haug, Aslaksen, & von Plessen, 2012). This can include re-evaluating and reframing goals

Figure 2.2 Single and Double Loop Organizational Learning

Single-Loop Learning
most common learning style,
problem solving

Governing Variables
Goals, values, beliefs,
conceptual frameworks

Why we do what we do

**Action Strategies
and Techniques**

What we do

**Results and
Consequences**

What we obtain

Double-Loop Learning
more than problem solving, this learning style
reevaluates and reframes goals, values, etc.

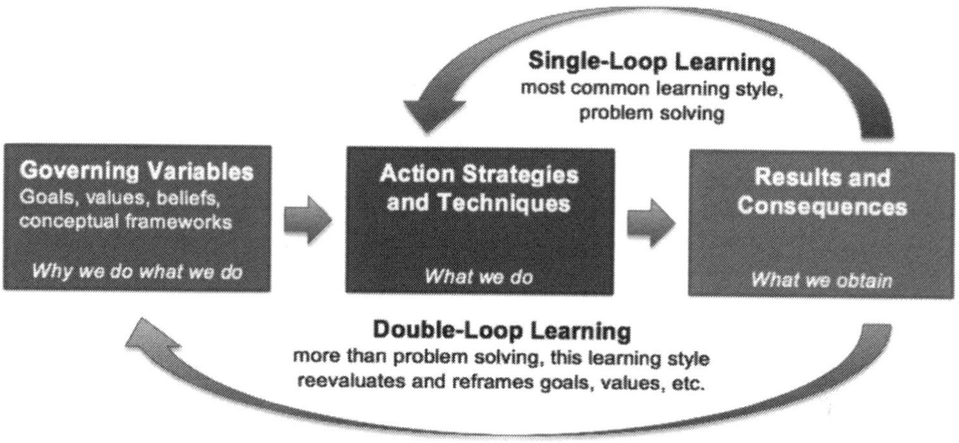

From www.afs.org/blog/icl/?p=2653

in the midst of a process improvement. Deep organizational change can involve a shift in individuals' shared mental models about the work being accomplished. In the complex adaptive health care environment, double-loop learning directs attention to the interdependency of processes and individuals, acknowledging the need to explore patterns of actions among these individuals (Hovlid et al., 2012). In the multi-disciplinary walkround example, double-loop learning might reveal conflicting belief systems among the disciplines as to the value of collaboration in infirmary care that is preventing implementation of the strategy.

The Learning Practice Program (LPP) proposes a practical method for increasing organizational learning. This model uses the action research cycle (Figure 2.3) to encourage organizational learning

Figure 2.3. Cycle of Action Research

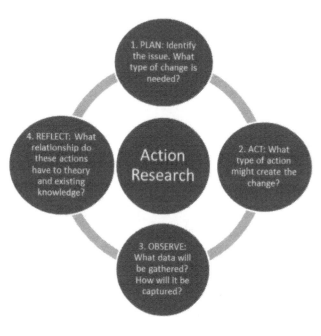

1. PLAN: Identify the issue. What type of change is needed?

2. ACT: What type of action might create the change?

3. OBSERVE: What data will be gathered? How will it be captured?

4. REFLECT: What relationship do these actions have to theory and existing knowledge?

Action Research

Adapted from Bunniss, et al., 2012

through quality improvement activities (Bunniss, Gray, & Kelly, 2012). This method has promise for use in the correctional setting. Using the Learning Practice Inventory as a diagnostic tool during intervals within the learning process, practice teams focus on quality initiatives while reflecting on individual and team learning moments (Rushmer et al., 2007). Participants value this active learning process for its effect on team communication, improvement in the quality of care provided by the group, and reduction of inter-professional barriers (Bunniss et al., 2012).

Summary

The unique nature of the correctional health care environment is an important consideration in efforts to reduce clinical error and improve patient safety. The blending of correctional and health care cultures can lead to friction and generate conflicting goals. Moving the organization from a culture of blame to a Just Culture can require great effort, involving the engagement of all levels within the organization and all health care disciplines. Leadership must play a major role in evaluating the culture, supporting staff as the second victim in a clinical error situation, and initiating safety culture best practices. Applying learning organization concepts enhances and accelerates movement to a safe and just environment of care.

References

Alert, S.E. (2008). Behaviors that undermine a culture of safety. *Sentinel Event Alert*, (40). Retrieved from http://ourpvh.com/docs/Disruptive_behavior/JCAHO-Behaviors_that_undermine_a_culture _of_safety.pdf

American Correctional Association (ACA). (1994). *ACA code of ethics.* Retrieved from http://www.aca.org/pastpresentfuture/ethics.asp

American Medical Association (AMA). (2008). *Model medical staff code of conduct.* Retrieved from www.ismanet.org/pdf/news/medicalstaffcodeofconduct.pdf

American Organization of Nurse Executives (AONE). (2005). *AONE guiding principles for excellence in nurse-physician relationships.* Retrieved from http://www.aone.org/resources/PDFs/AONE_GP_Excellence_Nurse_Physician.pdf

Barnsteiner, J.H. (2012). Safety. In G. Sherwood (Ed.), *Quality and safety in nursing: a competency approach to improving outcomes* (pp. 149–169). Chichester, West Sussex, UK: Wiley-Blackwell.

Bogue, B. & Cebula, N. (2012). *Applying the APEX assessment tools for organizational assessment.* Washington, DC: U.S. Department of Justice, National Institute of Corrections.

Bunniss, S., Gray, F., & Kelly, D. (2012). Collective learning, change and improvement in health care: Trialing a facilitated learning initiative with general practice teams: Facilitating shared learning in GP teams. *Journal of Evaluation in Clinical Practice*, 18(3), 630–636. doi:10.1111/j.1365-2753.2011.01641.x

Burhans, L.D., Chastain, K., & George, J. L. (2012). Just culture and nursing regulation: Learning to improve patient safety. *Journal of Nursing Regulation*, 2(4), 43–49.

Christensen, G. E. (2004). Leadership within corrections: The creation of learning organizations. *Corrections Managers' Report*, Feb/Mar, 55-56,66-67.

Claridge, T., Cook, G., & Hale, R. (2008). Organizational learning and patient safety in the NHS: An exploration of the organizational learning that occurs following a coroner's report under Rule 43. *Clinical Risk*, 14(1), 8-13. doi:10.1258/cr.2007.070001

Clochesy, J.M. (2008). The experience of diversity by generation: How to bridge the differences cohorts make up the US workforce. *The Diversity Factor*, 16(4), 15–19.

Colla, J.B. (2005). Measuring patient safety climate: A review of surveys. *Quality and Safety in Health Care*, 14(5), 364–366. doi:10.1136/qshc.2005.014217

Cumin, D., Boyd, M.J., Webster, C.S., & Weller, J.M. (2013). A systematic review of simulation for multidisciplinary team training in operating rooms. *Simulation in Healthcare: The Journal of the Society for Simulation in Healthcare*, 8(3), 171–179. doi:10.1097/SIH.0b013e31827e2f4c

Dekker, S. (2012). *Just culture: Balancing safety and accountability* (2nd edition). Surrey, England: Ashgate Publishing Limited.

Denham, C.R. (2007). TRUST: The 5 rights of the second victim. *Journal of Patient Safety, 3*(2), 107–119.

Edrees, H.H., Paine, L.A., Feroli, E.R., & Wu, A.W. (2011). Health care workers as second victims of medical errors. *Polskie Archiwum Medycyny Wewnetrznej, 121*(4), 101–108.

Emanuel, L., Berwick, D., Conway, J., Combes, J., Hatlie, M., Leape, L., ... Walton, M. (2008). What exactly is patient safety? *Advances in Patient Safety: New Directions and Alternative Approaches, 1.* Retrieved from http://ahrq.hhs. gov/downloads/pub/ advances2/vol1/Advances-Emanuel Berwick_110.pdf.

Fagan, M.J. (2012). Techniques to improve patient safety in hospitals. *JONA: The Journal of Nursing Administration, 42*(9), 426–430. doi:10.1097/NNA.0b013e3182664df5

Flin, R. (2010). Rudeness at work. *British Medical Journal, 340,* c2480–c2480. doi:10.1136/bmj.c2480

Frankel, A., Graydon-Baker, E., Neppl, C., Simmonds, T., Gustafson, M., & Gandhi, T.K. (2003). Patient safety leadership walkrounds. *Joint Commission Journal on Quality and Safety, 29*(1), 16–26.

Grissinger, M. (2011). Intimidation by superiors affects the safety of medical orders. *Pharmacy and Therapeutics, 36*(9), 544–563.

Hovlid, E., Bukve, O., Haug, K., Aslaksen, A. B., & von Plessen, C. (2012). Sustainability of healthcare improvement: What can we learn from learning theory? *BMC Health Services Research, 12*(1), 235.

Leape, L.L., Shore, M.F., Dienstag, J.L., Mayer, R.J., Edgman-Levitan, S., Meyer, G.S., & Healy, G.B. (2012). Perspective: A culture of respect, Part 2. *Academic Medicine, 87*(7), 853–858. doi:10.1097/ACM.0b013e3182583536

Marx, D. (2001). *Patient safety and the "Just Culture": A primer for healthcare executives.* New York, NY: Columbia University. Retrieved from www.safer.healthcare.ucla.edu/safer/archive/ahrq/FinalPrimerDoc.pdf

Morris, S. (2011). Just culture: Changing the environment of healthcare delivery. *Clinical Laboratory Science, 24*(2), 120–124.

National Commission on Correctional Health Care (NCCHC). (2014). *Standards for health services in prisons, 2014.* Chicago, IL: National Commission on Correctional Health Care.

National Institute of Corrections (NIC). (2014). *Establishing the learning organization e-course.* Retrieved from http://nicic.gov/training/nicwbt10

Nicholas, L. (2013). It's still a man's world...or is it? Advice for women working in corrections. *Corrections Today,* 41–44.

Nieva, V.F. & Sorra, J. (2003). Safety culture assessment: A tool for improving patient safety in healthcare organizations. *Quality and Safety in Health Care, 12*(suppl 2), ii17–ii23.

Painter, K. (2013). When doctors are bullies, patient safety may suffer. *USA Today,* April 30, 2013. Retrieved from www.usatoday.com/story/news/nation/ 2013/04/20/doctor-bullies-patients/2090995/

Pronovost, P. & Sexton, B. (2005). Assessing safety culture: Guidelines and recommendations. *Quality and Safety in Health Care, 14*(4), 231–233.

Rasmussen, J. (1982). Human errors: A taxonomy for describing human malfunction in industrial installations. *Journal of Occupational Accidents, 4*, 311–333.

Reason, J.T. (2008). *The human contribution: unsafe acts, accidents and heroic recoveries*. Farnham, England; Burlington, VT: Ashgate.

Rivard, P.E., Rosen, A.K., & Carroll, J.S. (2006). Enhancing patient safety through organizational learning: Are patient safety indicators a step in the right direction? *Health Services Research, 41*(4p2), 1633–1653. doi:10.1111/j.1475-6773.2006.00569.x

Rushmer, R.K., Kelly, D., Lough, M., Wilkinson, J.E., Greig, G.J., & Davies, H.T.O. (2007). The Learning Practice Inventory: Diagnosing and developing Learning Practices in the UK. *Journal of Evaluation in Clinical Practice, 13*(2), 206–211. doi:10.1111/j.1365-2753.2006.00673.x

Senge, P. (1990). *The fifth discipline.* London: Century Business.

Sexton, J.B., Helmreich, R.L., Neilands, T.B., Rowan, K., Vella, K., Boyden, J., & Thomas, E.J. (2006). The Safety Attitudes Questionnaire: Psychometric properties, benchmarking data, and emerging research. *BMC Health Services Research, 6*(1), 44.

Sportsman, S. & Hamilton, P. (2007). Conflict management styles in nursing and allied health professionals. *Journal of Professional Nursing, 23*(3), 157–166.

Stern, M.F., Greifinger, R.B., & Mellow, J. (2010). Patient safety: Moving the bar in prison health care standards. *American Journal of Public Health, 100*(11), 2103.

Agency for Healthcare Research and Quality. (2012). *Stories of success: Using CUSP to improve safety.* (2012, September 28). Retrieved July 30, 2013, from www.ahrq.gov/professionals/quality-patient-safety/cusp/cusp-success/index.html

Thomas, E.J., Sexton, J.B., Neilands, T.B., Frankel, A., & Helmreich, R.L. (2005). The effect of executive walk rounds on nurse safety climate attitudes: A randomized trial of clinical units. *BMC Health Services Research, 5*(1), 28.

Tucker, A.L. & Edmondson, A.C. (2003). Why hospitals don't learn from failures. *California Management Review, 45*(2), 55–72.

Wachter, R.M. (2012). Understanding patient safety (2nd ed.). New York, NY: Mcgraw-Hill.

Wagner, L.M., Capezuti, E., & Rice, J. C. (2009). Nurses' perceptions of safety culture in long-term care settings. Journal of Nursing Scholarship, 41(2), 184–192. doi:10.1111/j.1547-5069.2009.01270.x

Watts, B.V., Percarpio, K., West, P., & Mills, P.D. (2010). Use of the Safety Attitudes Questionnaire as a measure in patient safety improvement. *Journal of Patient Safety, 6*(4), 206–209.

Weaver, S.J., Lubomksi, L.H., Wilson, R.F., Pfoh, E.R., Martinez, K.A., & Dy, S.M. (2013). Promoting a culture of safety as a patient safety strategy: A systematic review. *Annals of Internal Medicine, 158*(5_Part_2), 369–374.

3 Systems for Therapeutic Action

Patient care is delivered within a complex system of interacting components that affect the process and outcome of care. These interacting components have weaknesses that lead to clinical errors. Vulnerabilities within the system of care delivery, including the potential for miscommunication among staff and patients, create an ongoing need for attention to improve patient safety. This can be especially concerning in correctional health care where practitioners must effectively practice within the criminal justice system among many disciplines. This increases the number of interacting components for standard processes and adds barriers to care delivery.

Systems of care, then, are an important component of a patient safety environment (Figure 3.1). Therapeutic systems, based on principles of high reliability systems design and human factors engineering, reduce the potential for patient harm. Communication and teamwork based on transdisciplinary collaboration can stabilize communication patterns to improve patient safety within this system (Table 3.1).

Figure 3.1 A Patient Safety Model of Health Care

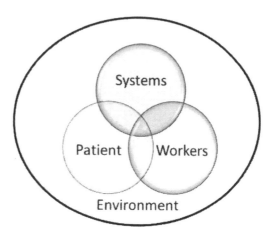

Adapted from Emanuel et al., 2008

High Reliability Systems Design

Complex organizations with potential for great human mortality, such as chemical processing plants, air traffic control, and nuclear power plants, must anticipate the worst and be equipped to prevent and handle it. Over time, these industries have designed high reliability systems to prevent error and improve safety (Reason, 2000). These high reliability organizations develop predictable and effective operations, greatly reducing hazards that could harm many individuals (Carroll & Rudolph, 2006). Health care systems are applying principles from other high reliability organization disciplines to reduce patient harm.

There are many similarities between health care delivery and these high reliability industries. The dynamic interplay of system, process, and individual practices must be continually fine-tuned in the midst of active

Table 3.1. Domains and Principles of Patient Safety

Domain of Patient Safety	Principle of Patient Safety
Environment of Care	A Just Culture in a Learning Organization
Systems for Therapeutic Action	High Reliability System Design Communication and Teamwork
Recipient of Care	Patient-Centered Care
Health Care Workers	Competent Care Providers Communication and Teamwork

engagement. Participants in the process are making small adjustments along the continuum to invisibly affect the outcome. Frequent and routine interruptions must be continually managed. Interruptions can come from many sources. In the correctional setting, distractions such as unexpected intakes, security requests, lockdowns, and yard brawls vie for staff attention along with standard patient care needs. The organization must be designed with system controls and governance to accommodate a duality of "standardization with flexibility, conformity with initiative, accountability with learning, anticipation with resilience, cost reduction with safety" (Carroll & Rudolph, 2006, p. i5).

Challenges in High Reliability Organizations

Hines, Luna, Loftus, Marquardt & Stelmokas (2008) describe the challenges of health care organizations that parallel high reliability organizations and, therefore, justify the use of high reliability system design in a health care setting. These commonalities are described in Table 3.2.

Many characteristics of high reliability organizations apply to the health care setting. The human variability of care provider and patient adds to the complexity and requires contextual consideration in applying high reliability industry principles. "We don't make widgets" is a phrase that exemplifies the differences between health care and more automated industries. Although every industry deals with the frailties of human operators, health care also deals with the complex interaction of patient and disease. The objective of the organization – patient healing – involves the interaction of a unique individual's response to one or more acute or chronic conditions. This adds unpredictability to the system (Hines et al., 2008). Patient unpredictability, coupled with the individual care and treatment preferences of providers, escalates variability within the system. This variability is also increased by the high mobility of the health care workforce. Periods of particularly rapid staff turnover can add significant risk to a complex care delivery system (Hines et al., 2008).

Table 3.2 Common Challenges in High Reliability Organizations

Challenge	Description
Hyper-complexity	Multi-team systems must be coordinated for safety
Tight Coupling	Team members depend on task completion by other team members in order to function
Extreme Hierarchical Differentiation	Highly structured and differentiated roles within the team
Multiple Decision-makers in a Complex Communication Network	Many interconnected decisions combine to deliver service requiring a complex communication network
High Degree of Accountability	Each staff member has accountability for their part of a process that risks error affecting one or more patients
Need for Frequent, Immediate Feedback	Decision-making within the system is affected by ever-changing circumstances which require constant feedback
Compressed Time Constraints	Patient outcomes are affected by timing of decisions and actions

Adapted from Hines, et al., 2008; Roberts & Rousseau, 1989

High Reliability Organization Principles

So, how can high reliability organization principles be applied to the correctional health care setting? High reliability organizations create a collective mindfulness around safety that consists of five qualities: sensitivity to operations, reluctance to simplify, preoccupation with failure, deference to expertise, and resilience (Hines et al., 2008). As these qualities of safety mindfulness are developed in individuals and collectively within the correctional health care setting, patient safety is improved and clinical error decreased.

Sensitivity to operations. Sensitivity to operations is described as an active mindset of both leadership and staff toward the current state of systems and processes of care. Once a process is established, it is easy to degenerate due to staff work-arounds, changes in other tangential and overlapping processes (such as custody schedules), and staff turnover. High reliability organizations continually "mind" the systems and processes that are in place to determine if they are being followed, pick up the pieces if they are not, and consider improvements if they are no longer working well. Sensitivity to operations also involves an understanding of circumstances that can affect outcomes such as team member fatigue, distraction, variability of workload, and resource availability (McKeon, Oswaks, & Cunningham, 2006).

Reluctance to simplify. Though simplifying processes in a complex and chaotic environment can be helpful, focusing on the simplest answer to an issue is not. High reliability organizations understand that the complexity of interaction within the work setting requires strategies for gathering all information to make an informed decision about the cause of a clinical error and the most effective course of action to improve patient safety. Oversimplification of adverse events can lead to a shallow interpretation of the root cause and subsequently a Band-Aid approach to system correction.

Technology is a tempting area of process simplification that can cause as many problems as it eliminates (Dekker, 2011). An electronic medical record (EMR) can be viewed as automating many documentation chores that are time-consuming, repetitive, and lack standardization across patients and practitioners. Adding any technology to a system also adds new work and skill requirements, however, that can offset any work reductions gained through automation. High reliability organizations understand that technology may add more complexity than simplicity to a care environment and, therefore, accommodate for appropriate staff education and process integration when adding new technology.

Preoccupation with failure. Some organizational cultures may see the prevention of an error as an indication of success. High reliability organizations see near misses as opportunities to adjust a faulty system or process for improvement before a catastrophe happens (Hines et al., 2008). Mindfulness of failure potential is encouraged to reduce staff complacency (Spath, 2011). Without constant reminders, humans develop a tolerance for risk. Reminders and tools can keep fear of error ever-present.

Deference to expertise. In a highly differentiated organizational structure, deference to expertise – no matter the level – leads to the most knowledgeable and skilled individual making important decisions. Leaders in High reliability organizations listen to clinical experts at every level in determining a course of action. With all team members sensitive to potential system failure and leaders open to the input of all, even "weak signal" system faults can be identified and rectified prior to a catastrophic event (McKeon et al., 2006). This de-emphasis on hierarchy and emphasis on open communication allows each team member to fully contribute to patient safety from their own professional perspective (Hines et al., 2008). For example, correctional health care and custody leadership often work together on combined efforts such as an influenza outbreak or a disaster response. Each profession contributes expertise to manage the priorities and a successful resolution often hinges on open communication among them.

Resilience. A resilient organization prepares for the worst at all times. This can include frequent simulations, such as disaster drills, or prospective risk evaluations (Spath, 2011). In addition, a resilient organization allows team members to make immediate course adjustments when system failures emerge. Team members are capable of improvising to contain errors (Hines et al., 2008). This could mean shifting personnel and resources to the area of need, such as a large influx of detainees requiring intake screening. High reliability organization team members are ever-mindful that systems can fail in unanticipated ways that require creative solutions.

These five characteristics of corporate mindfulness in an organization lead to reduction in error and increased safety. Their primary focus is on the blunt end of error reduction: altering upstream system factors before a significant error emerges. This mindfulness allows the collective organization to work toward draining the swamp as a solution to mosquito infestation rather than each individual continuing to swat their own tormentors (Reason, 2000).

Human Factor Engineering

Highly reliable systems require attention to the human factors that affect error. Human factors engineering involves coordinating the interaction of humans, equipment, technology, and environment with a goal of designing a system that provides safeguards or barriers to common human error (Wachter, 2012). Human factor engineering, then, is a user-centered system design process that maximizes an understanding of human capabilities and limitations to alter work components for safe outcomes (Gosbee, 2002).

Spath (2011) has organized common human factor engineering concepts from the High reliability organization literature that are most effective when applied to the health care setting. They are explained here with examples for the correctional setting.

Reduce Reliance on Memory

Memory can fail us, especially when we are preoccupied with juggling multiple changing priorities. Human factor engineering principles reduce the need for memory in key safety situations. Memory is also a concern when important tasks or situations are infrequent yet complicated. Checklists and written protocols are safety mechanisms to reduce reliance on memory. For example, a written alcohol withdrawal protocol assures that care providers consider every angle in deciding about monitoring, medication administration, and housing.

Requiring recognition of what to do rather than relying on recall is advantageous when memories are overloaded (Wachter, 2012). Recognizing a list of conditions to consider when assessing diffuse abdominal pain in a sick call situation is safer than expecting the nurse to remember all the conditions that might generate such a symptom. Reducing the reliance on memory and decreasing the need for prolonged vigilance are user-centered design principles (Barnsteiner, 2012).

> *"Most providers in corrections are generalists, so using recall and having all of the requisite knowledge needed for complex clinical situations is impossible. Human error is more likely when medical information resources are not available during clinic time. Access to physician resources in Oregon is easy in that the DOC has invested in top-notch internet resources and cell phones for most providers. We believe this provides an effective strategy for improved care and decreased risk. Many systems, fearing security or cost issues, will not allow internet access "inside"- Oregon has managed to do so safely and cost-effectively. Clearly, given the will, other systems can safely do the same."*
> **– Mike Puerini, MD, CCHP-A, Salem, Oregon, Immediate Past President, Society of Correctional Physicians**

Remaining vigilant for long periods of time is also a safety concern. Vigilance is important when required to monitor patients for suicide and self-injury. Even with checklists, staff can become complacent or mentally fatigued over long periods of time. Rotating staff assignments and scheduling breaks throughout the shift can decrease failing vigilance (Barnsteiner, 2012).

Alarms are another way to improve vigilance. Medication delivery devices such as IV pumps have alarm systems that stop action until user input is provided. In busy infirmaries, staff may override sensitive alarm systems to avoid the increased noise in a chaotic environment. This dangerous practice can increase error (Graham & Cvach, 2010); better to calibrate the alarm system to meet the individual needs of the patient and situation. Of course, staff must be able to hear alarms when they sound. Heavy cell doors and nursing station locations can reduce sound transmission in an infirmary environment. Those patients receiving high-risk treatments need to be within sight and sound of a nurse at all times.

Improve Information Access

Safe and appropriate clinical decision-making is more likely if information is available at the point of care (Spath, 2011). In technology-rich environments, this can include electronic access to drug information, decision trees, and treatment protocols. The constraints of the correctional health care environment must be taken into consideration in applying this principle. Still, written aids such as dosage conversion charts on the medication cart, resuscitation protocols on the code cart, and sick call protocols in the treatment room can greatly improve patient safety.

Mistake-Proof Processes

Human factor engineering design involves the inclusion of error barriers within clinical processes. This can include a forced function, which is a design feature that requires a specific action before the next step in a process can be performed (Wachter, 2012). A forced function might be as simple as having only one nurse with the keys to open a locked drawer before administering a narcotic. Alarms and shutdowns of equipment, such as security entrances, are also examples of forced function that can improve safety (Reason, 2000). Electronic medical records may require specific data entry before allowing the ordering of a lethal drug (Spath, 2011).

Unit and System Design

Poorly designed systems or work environments encourage staff work-arounds to deliver necessary care. A common example in correctional health care is the practice of borrowing medications from one patient's supply to provide to another patient when their medication is missing. Another example might be the frequent practice of pre-pouring medications to work around a care environment with hallways too narrow for medication carts or the need to use stairwells to access patients.

Surprisingly, the ability to get the job done in the face of a dysfunctional system is often a prized skill in health care, although work-arounds can also lead to errors when they involve short-circuiting necessary safety steps.

The chaotic correctional environment adds noise and distraction that can affect the accuracy of important care tasks such as medication administration. Alteration in system design can reduce distractions and interruptions to improve clinician concentration. Studies show that simple interventions such as "quiet zone" signage or medication administration vests reduce interruptions by providing a visual cue that nurses are engaged in high-concentration activities (Klejka, 2012; Rivera & Karsh, 2010).

Standardize Tasks

Repetitive tasks that must be done by many individuals within a workgroup can be standardized for consistency and error reduction. Task standardization also creates a structure for process movement. For example, use of the Subjective-Objective-Assessment-Plan (SOAP) structure in a nursing sick call protocol can standardize the assessment and intervention process by guiding the nurse through the subjective and objective assessments necessary to make an appropriate clinical judgment and treatment decision.

The use of standard clinical guidelines for disease treatment also contributes to patient safety. Although care providers still consider individual patient's needs, use of these guidelines standardizes practice and assures attention to all aspects of the condition.

Reduce the Number of Hand-offs

Interdependency among groups is a factor of High reliability organizations that requires close attention to the hand-off process. Weak links in the communication chain can lead to clinical error; therefore, the smallest number of hand-offs possible is recommended to reduce the number of opportunities for missed communication of important information (Carroll & Rudolph, 2006). As additional hand-offs are added to a clinical process, complexity and opportunities for missed information also increases. Decreasing the number of hand-offs in corrections can include the use of telemedicine for specialist visits and use of team reporting rather than same discipline (nurse-to-nurse or physician-to-physician) reporting. Telemedicine, in particular, can reduce hand-offs when the ordering practitioner sits in on the telemedicine visit.

In the correctional setting, patients are frequently sent out for specialist evaluations and treatments. Outgoing officer transport must include medical records, and the receiving staff must communicate the evaluation information back to the primary provider for ongoing management. Every hand-off of the patient and patient information in this progression has potential for lost information. When hand-offs cannot be reduced, correctional health care experts recommend systems to track specialist consults and diagnostic testing to be sure that critical communication is reviewed and acted upon (Stern, Greifinger, & Mellow, 2010).

Communication, Collaboration, and Teamwork

Correctional health care is a complex adaptive system within the criminal justice system. Embedded and nested teams must communicate and collaborate to accomplish mutual goals. Formal and informal communication structures and processes foster effective communication among and within various disciplines and teams, which involves navigation through various people, politics, and culture (Carroll & Rudolph, 2006). Communication is more than verbal and written words, as it encompasses the body language, attitude, and voice tone of both sender and receiver (Nadzam, 2009). Effective communication requires the foundation of a supportive organizational and clinical culture described in Chapter 2, as well as an understanding of the effects of the organization, environment, and individual on the message sent and received.

Communication

It is well-known that communication failures are a frequent cause of clinical error and a frequent component of medical malpractice claims (World Health Organization, 2007). A Joint Commission analysis of data spanning 10 years showed miscommunication as a leading cause of sentinel events in the acute care setting (TJC, 2013). Understanding the factors affecting clinical communication and initiating steps to improve communication among care providers can reduce error. Factors are categorized into three areas: organizational, environmental and individual.

Organizational. As described in Chapter 2, incivility in the workplace can be a barrier to open clinical communication. If an organization turns a blind eye to episodes of incivility, poor interpersonal behavior gains a stronghold and discourages both standard clinical communication and the special communication needed when patient safety is in jeopardy. Intervening during a potential error can be personally and professionally risky. Many clinicians desire to avoid confrontation and will seek out other means, or just let go of a concern, rather than risk speaking up.

Besides incivility, an organizational culture that does not want to hear bad news, or punishes those who bring it, will not encourage the free communication needed to prevent or interrupt an unsafe situation. A management culture that encourages covering up errors (or even potential errors) can be dangerous to both patients and staff. Unfortunately, this type of culture is inherent in many correctional systems.

Communication is built on relationships (Manning, 2006). Organizations that support and encourage respectful interpersonal relationships among all staff members provide a foundation for effective communication. Organizations that support and encourage hierarchy and social structure provide a barrier to communication. Correctional settings are often steeped in hierarchy and protocol that can thwart the interpersonal relationships that encourage open communication.

Environmental. The care delivery environment has a significant effect on the ability to communicate. The communication process is complex and involves listening, assimilating, interpreting, discriminating, gathering, and sharing information (Manning, 2006). Difficult at the best of times, communication can be nearly impossible in the hectic, noisy, interruption-filled correctional health care setting. Effort must go toward reducing the distractions and interruptions that plague the environment of care.

Correctional health care units, particularly in older facilities, may have been an afterthought in design. Practitioners, therefore, must 'make do' in a less-than-optimal

> "Correctional health care presents a rapid turnover of patients and a frequently chaotic atmosphere. Jails, especially, can be compared to city emergency rooms - with a plethora of diagnoses and multiple patients arriving together. During the more hectic periods, whether in small jails or large, medical staff are tasked to keep track of all arriving detainees, in order to provide intake screening in a small window of time. Communication between medical staff and correctional staff is critical, but not always smooth. In a large jail, patients can be "lost" without this critical component of care. Very ill patients can be lost in the system, i.e. forgotten and not assessed within prescribed windows, due to failure of security and nursing staff to communicate between shifts. The implementation of "huddles" at change of shift would have prevented this error. A patient suffered serious issues with detoxification and medical complications, due to lack of this type of communication. In addition to improving communication, these huddles improved teamwork among staff and security."
> **– Johnnie R. Lambert, RN, CCHP, Licensed Healthcare Risk Manager, Beaufort, NC**

physical environment. Physical barriers can easily become communication barriers when team members are separated by locked doors or located in different buildings on the grounds. Medical and mental health practitioners, for example, are more likely to have spontaneous face-to-face interactions if their work spaces are joined. Likewise, physicians and nurses are more likely to collaborate if there is easy access among their clinical spaces.

In the correctional environment, team members frequently communicate in writing or by phone. This can lead to misinterpretation of information or missing information needed for effective decision-making. Staff may need to contact multiple providers in various locations to establish a plan of care for a complex patient situation. Various fragmented communications, along with time constraints and a heavy workload, can lead to missed information Team members must seek out ways to reduce these communication barriers such as establishing no-interruption communication periods or using door-closed times for high-priority communications.

Individual. Characteristics of the individuals involved in communication, whether staff or patient, can also affect the outcome. Although a communication episode can be dissected into three parts – the sender, the message, and the receiver – each part is complex. Whether the individual is the sender or the receiver, various characteristics can affect the outcome such as these proposed by O'Daniel and Rosenstein (2008).

- Personal values and expectations
- Personality differences
- Hierarchy
- Disruptive behavior
- Culture and ethnicity
- Generational differences
- Gender
- Differences in language and jargon
- Varying levels of preparation, qualifications and status

Cultural differences among team members can affect the nature, delivery, and understanding of the message. In addition, language fluency and accent can confuse interpretation. Culture can affect the willingness of the individual to openly challenge a decision or action (O'Daniel & Rosenstein, 2008). Indirect communication in this regard can be easily missed by the receiver. In addition, culture can ascribe specific meaning to non-verbal communication such as facial expression and voice tone.

The effect of differences in socioeconomic status among team members is often underestimated. Staff members from perceived lower statuses who see an error by a perceived higher-status individual may be reluctant to bring it to their attention. Likewise, individuals with low literacy skills may not ask clarification questions and rely on assumptions rather than be perceived as ignorant or slow (Woods, 2006).

Gender plays a role in clinical communication with women. Older women, in particular, tend to provide more detailed backgrounds and attach more affect to the interaction (Elderkin-Thompson & Waitzkin, 1999). This can make prioritizing information difficult. Gender can also cloud communication with sexual innuendo or overtones, real or imagined.

Personality characteristics, especially demeaning behaviors such as condescension, intimidation, and abusive language, can hamper effective clinical communication. Approachability is an important factor in the determination to initiate a difficult discussion. Bullying in the workplace, when tolerated and even engrained in the culture, leads to "work-around" maneuvering to avoid the abusive individual, thus hindering effective communication and leading to clinical error. Bullying may also lead to depression, fear, anxiety, and isolation that hinder good clinical decision-making (Murray, 2009).

Nurses prefer to either avoid or accommodate others in a potential conflict (Sportsman & Hamilton, 2007). In an oppressive environment, nurses are more likely to avoid and accommodate poor behavior rather than address it (Sayre, McNeese-Smith, Leach, & Phillips, 2012); but this silence can be deadly. A study of 1,700 health care staff in 13 urban, suburban, and rural hospitals found that more than half of the participants had witnessed coworkers cutting corners, breaking rules, or demonstrating incompetence without speaking up about it (Maxwell, Grenny, McMillan, Patterson, & Switzler, 2005).

Individuals who know, like, and trust each other can sometimes overcome the personal characteristics of sender and receiver. Conversely, clinical communication among unfamiliar parties can lead to assumptions, misinterpretation of intent, and risk-averse responses. For example, an on-call physician, unfamiliar with the patient in question and the nurse calling about the patient's chest pain, may choose to send the patient out to the emergency room rather than trust the nurse's assessment findings or EKG abilities. Likewise, a nurse who has been demeaned in the past by a fellow nurse may be hesitant to request assistance with a challenging patient situation. Actions to encourage knowing, liking, and trusting team members enhance approachability and encourage effective communication. Team members value familiarity over formality in health care interactions (O'Daniel & Rosenstein, 2008).

It can be difficult to sort out the causes of a communication failure. Manning (2006) suggests three primary categories of clinical communication failure based on the work of Reason (1997). The categories of system, message, and recipient failures can guide the analysis of a clinical error that holds a communication component (Table 3.3).

Table 3.3 Communication Failure Categories

Failure Type	Cause
System	Channels of communication did not exist or were not functioning
Message	Necessary information was not transmitted
Reception	Information was misinterpreted by the recipient

Adapted from Manning, 2006

Interdisciplinary Collaboration

While effective communication involves the exchange of information between sender and receiver, collaboration builds on a communication base to use the information to cooperatively work together, share responsibility for problem-solving, and make mutually agreed-upon decisions (O'Daniel & Rosenstein, 2008). Interdisciplinary collaboration is the most frequently used term for collaboration among the various disciplines within health care to affect patient care outcomes; however, the term transdisciplinary collaboration is gaining popularity as a more accurate description of the concept.

Petri's (2010) concept analysis of interdisciplinary collaboration in health care noted three primary attributes: problem-focused, sharing, and working together. Interdisciplinary collaboration focuses on solving problems surrounding a patient situation through various interactive modes. This is accomplished through shared responsibility and decision-making in a cooperative context. By working together in a complementary fashion, each discipline is able to bring their unique perspective to bear on the situation, contributing to a better outcome than any single discipline might effect.

In correctional health care delivery, interdisciplinary collaboration extends to include custody frontline staff and management. The intertwined practices of health care and custody require the same principles of collaborative practice to accomplish mutual goals and to resolve conflict when competing goals are present. Active and open communication between health care and correctional staff is essential to optimal operations. Accreditation standards encourage interdisciplinary collaboration, particularly at the administrative level and when dealing with the special needs inmates who may require additional medical attention, special housing, or use of medical equipment in their living area (NCCHC, 2014).

Benefits of collaboration. The body of evidence is growing that interdisciplinary collaboration improves patient safety and positive clinical outcomes. Lack of interdisciplinary collaboration can be frustrating to care providers, but it has also been linked to increased clinical error. O'Daniel and Rosenstein (2008) found evidence of a relationship between interdisciplinary collaboration and reduced medication errors, risk of inpatient mortality, and shorter hospitals stays. Improving collaboration among health professionals, and between health care professionals and correctional staff, then, could significantly reduce legal risk and improve patient safety.

Petri (2010) analyzed the consequences of interdisciplinary collaboration and found that collaboration enhanced coordination of services and promotion of holistic care in a fragmented care system. Improving collaboration in correctional health care, then, would be important to the efficiency of care delivery. Interdisciplinary collaboration also improves productivity and cost containment.

Barriers to collaboration. Many barriers to effective collaboration among disciplines in non-correctional practice settings can be acute in the correctional setting. The episodic and transient nature of health care delivery in a correctional setting can decrease the ability of team members to develop trusting, cohesive relationships. Smaller correctional settings may need to cobble together health care teams consisting of part-time on-site staff and on-call providers from the community. Even larger systems may rotate on-call staff across several facilities so that the weekend provider may not know the patient population or facilities' standards. High staff turnover or vacancy rates can lead to use of agency and travel staff with unknown skills and abilities. These are just some of the realities of correctional health care that can lead to a lack of trust.

Lack of trust is a barrier to interdisciplinary collaboration (McKeon et al., 2006). Trusting, cohesive relationships are necessary for multiple disciplines to be willing to consider differing viewpoints on a situation and negotiate a satisfying solution. Role clarification and role valuing will help develop trust that leads to truly listening to the perspective of other disciplines.

The lack of a shared worldview among the disciplines in a correctional facility also discourages collaboration (McKeon et al., 2006; Nadzam, 2009). Discipline-specific viewpoints on the goals of patient care can make collaboration difficult if team members cannot channel the diversity of perspectives toward productive use. Team members must learn to see different perspectives as enhancing care provision rather than feeling a need to dismiss or discourage a variety of goals. Remaining patient-centered in the collaboration process helps overcome conflicting worldviews (AONE, 2005).

Hierarchy differences, actual and perceived, can be a barrier to collaboration. Power and status differentials must be minimized to encourage collaborative activities, especially the involvement of those in traditionally lower statuses (Sayre et al., 2012). Organizational structures that leave lower-status staff playing a subservient role can hinder the peer relationship necessary for open dialog. Without an organizational culture advocating collaborative practice, correctional health care professionals struggling to meet time demands may see little need to engage the viewpoints of other disciplines (including security staff) in the decision-making process (Fewster-Thuente & Velsor-Friedrich, 2008).

Lack of time, in fact, can be a huge deterrent to interdisciplinary collaboration. Various disciplines, managing patient care needs episodically and at different times of the day or week, may have little opportunity to discuss a challenging patient situation. Communication may be limited to reviewing and responding to individual team member notes or brief phone contacts.

Developing collaboration among disciplines. Correctional health care organizations desiring to improve interdisciplinary collaboration can first look to eliminating the barriers of trust, shared worldview, hierarchical differences, and time pressures in the clinical setting. In addition, several specific interventions for improving interdisciplinary collaboration show promising results.

Interdisciplinary education is commonly noted to improve collaboration (AONE, 2005; Disch, 2012; Interprofessional Education Collaborative Expert Panel, 2011; Petri, 2010). Although most advantageous during pre-professional education, interdisciplinary education can be helpful at any time. Holding joint grand rounds, conducting monthly educational meetings for all disciplines, and using CQI and M&M reviews as an interdisciplinary educational opportunity are ways to accomplish interdisciplinary education in the correctional setting.

Interdisciplinary rounding can be effective for improving collaboration among the professions (Fewster-Thuente & Velsor-Friedrich, 2008). A rounding structure provides a framework of patient-centered dialog among the disciplines. Rounding allows for setting short and long-term patient goals and provides a platform for negotiation of any competing goals among the respective disciplinary perspectives. They could be adapted for use in an infirmary, or virtual rounding could take place during an interdisciplinary team meeting.

Role awareness among the security and health care professions improves collaboration by clearing away role ambiguity among team participants (Arford, 2005;

Petri, 2010). An understanding of each team member's role encourages trust and role valuing. Understanding the knowledge, skills, and perspectives of each discipline in the team clarifies roles and establishes the need for participative decision-making.

Taking deliberate action to support and encourage collaboration is needed for it to become a reality (Petri, 2010). Without focused attention on developing skills and organizational expectations for collaboration among the disciplines in a correctional setting, mitigating circumstance will effectively eliminate the behavior. Organizational leaders must foster collaboration and develop a structure to support the ongoing practice of this discipline.

Teamwork

Communication and collaboration are foundational to quality teamwork. Individual member skills in communicating and collaborating among team members enhance teamwork. While collaboration and teamwork are often used synonymously, the concepts have important differences. In analyzing the concept of teamwork, Xyrichis and Ream (2008) found this term strongly emphasized an interdependence that was much more than merely collaboration. With concerted effort, teams achieve patient-centered goals through interdependent collaboration and shared decision-making. This requires team members to understand and enact their professional roles to meet common health goals (Xyrichis & Ream, 2008).

Teamwork contributes to the prevention of adverse events (Manser, 2009). To move a work group from merely a team of experts to an expert team requires specific group skills development (Baker, Gustafson, Beaubien, Salas, & Barach, 2005; Burke, 2004). Team performance success factors include these suggested by O'Daniel and Rosenstein (2008).

- Clear direction
- Clear and known roles and tasks for team members
- Shared responsibility for team success
- Appropriate balance of member participation for the task at hand
- Acknowledgment and processing of conflict
- Clear specifications regarding authority and accountability
- Clear and known decision-making procedures
- Regular and routine communication sharing
- Access to needed resources
- Mechanism to evaluate outcomes and adjust accordingly

A major theme in this listing is the need for clarity of structure, process, and expected outcome in team functioning. Without clear direction, roles, task, or authority, a team can flounder in meeting patient care goals. Lack of conflict processing, decision-making procedures and communication channels also decrease team functioning. Without a structured mechanism for outcome evaluation and team feedback, group learning and improvement is lacking.

Teamwork dimensions. High functioning teams coordinate, communicate, and share responsibility through an interrelated process of five dimensions (Figure 3.2). First, they create and maintain a team climate and structure. Within that structure, the team plans and problem-solves while communicating and managing the team workload. They regularly review the outcome of teamwork to consider how to improve teamwork skills over time (Riser, Simon, Rice, Mary L. Salisbury, & Morey, 2011).

Figure 3.2. Interrelationships of the Five Team Dimensions

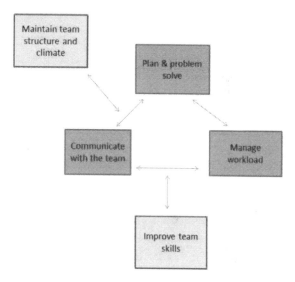

Adapted from Riser, Simon, Rice, Salisbury, & Morey, 2011, p. 308

Developing Teamwork Skills

Most clinical professions focus on developing individual skills during pre-licensure education; therefore, many clinicians come to the correctional health care team with some rudimentary ability in communication and collaboration activities without true skill in working among multiple disciplines as a team. Teamwork skill development, then, must be a focus of professional development activities in the correctional setting. Several team training frameworks, developed and advocated for the traditional health care setting, have application in correctional health care.

TeamSTEPPS Training System

One training program gaining popularity and showing evidence of improving patient safety is the Team Strategies and Tools to Enhance Performance and Patient Safety (TeamSTEPPS) training program developed by the Department of Defense (DoD) and the Agency for Healthcare Research and Quality (AHRQ). In use since 2006, this training program focuses on core teamwork skills of leadership, communication, situation

Figure 3.3 TeamSTEPPS

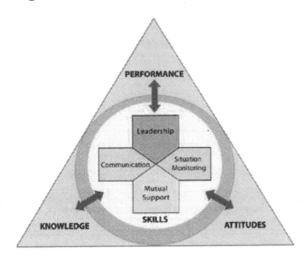

AHRQ. Public Domain

monitoring, and mutual support (AHRQ, 2010). Figure 3.3 provides a visual representation of the interaction of these four skills in team implementation. TeamSTEPPS is a structured training program that teaches necessary teamwork skills in a succinct manner and provides the tools for teams to be successful.

The effect of team training can be difficult to quantify, but evidence is building that the TeamSTEPPS structured training program increases patient safety. For example, one hospital reduced medication error by 30% and patient falls by 88% after implementing training for all staff members (Healthcare Risk Management, 2012). A review of research on TeamSTEPPS implementation found improved operating room functioning with reduced retained instruments and error rates (Coburn & Gage-Croll, 2011).

TeamSTEPPS training provides a shared mental model for team members. To work as a cohesive team, members must learn team leadership processes for planning, problem-solving, and process

Table 3.4. DESC Conflict Management Script

Script Component	Description
D	Describe the specific situation
E	Express your concerns about the action
S	Suggest other alternatives
C	Consequences should be stated

From AHRQ, 2010

improvement. Structured communications around these areas include briefings for planning, huddles for problem-solving, and debriefs for process improvement reviews (Ferguson, 2008). The shared mental model of TeamSTEPPS allows situation monitoring among team members. Members actively monitor the actions of other team members in a mutually respectful and accountable fashion. Monitoring identifies a need to share workload to reduce or avoid errors. This encourages mutual support among team members. Support is provided through tools such as the two-challenge rule, where a team member must voice a concern at least twice, and the DESC script (Table 3.4), which provides a constructive approach to conflict management (AHRQ, 2010). Specific team communication tools include SBAR, call-out, check-back and hand-off (Table 3.5).

Crew Resource Management (CRM)

Originating in the aviation industry to standardize communication and teamwork for improved safety (O'Daniel & Rosenstein, 2008), this training program uses simulation and interactive group debriefings to strengthen teamwork. CRM is a framework on which the TeamSTEPPS program was built. Competence is developed in six key areas: managing fatigue, creating and managing teams, recognizing adverse situations, crosschecking and communication, decision making and performance feedback (Disch, 2012).

Table 3.5. TeamSTEPPS Communication Tools

Tool	Description
SBAR	Structured communication with linear progression of information: Situation, Background, Assessment, Recommendation.
Call-Out	Critical information request in an emergency situation such as resuscitation.
Check-Back	Confirming communication has been accurately received by having receiver repeat back the information.
Hand-off	Structured passing on of information and responsibility for a patient.

Adapted from Ferguson, 2008

Dynamic decision-making necessary in aviation is similar to that of many health care settings (Disch, 2012), although evidence is mixed on the outcome of CRM team training in health care. A review of the literature found that a pediatric setting increased perceived team collaboration following implementation, while a surgical setting felt little change in team compliance with perioperative safety practices

(Fagan, 2012). Adaptations of CRM concepts to the health care setting may be a reason that the TeamSTEPPS education program is showing more positive results.

Team Skill Development Follow-Up Actions

Structured follow-up activities have been found to improve team development. Several specific follow-up activities are recommended to improve communication and follow-through.

Debriefing. Regular debriefing exercises can strengthen team skills while overcoming barriers to success (Wachter, 2012). The outcome of debriefing sessions, however, relies on the team members' ability to remain open to change and reduce defensiveness or accusation in the process. Debriefing sessions should be as blame-free as possible and focus on the learning potential of every sentinel event or near-miss event (O'Daniel & Rosenstein, 2008).

Team failure checklist. An extension of the debriefing process is the use of structured teamwork evaluation tools such as the Teamwork Failure Checklist. After a significant incident, team members evaluate team functioning across the five team dimensions of Figure 3.3 by responding to various questions. Then, team members assess the impact of effective teamwork on the outcome of the incident by determining if teamwork may have prevented or mitigated the occurrence (Riser et al., 2011).

A systematic review of evidence for various patient safety strategies strongly encourages team training (Shekelle et al., 2013). Correctional settings can benefit from targeted team training in principles found in the CRM or TeamSTEPPS programs, even if they do not adapt the full structured program.

Structures that Encourage Communication

Structures that encourage communication are a major part of systems for therapeutic action. Several structured communication elements have been found to reduce clinical error and improve patient safety. Implementing these structures in the correctional clinical setting can provide stability to clinical communication processes.

Checklists

The patient safety movement has embraced checklists since research on the use of checklists to reduce surgical error showed startling results (Semel et al., 2010). Working with the World Health Organization (WHO), researchers implemented a simple pre-surgical checklist in eight hospitals and found a 36% decrease in major post-operative complications and a 47% decrease in post-operative mortality. Since then, WHO has developed checklists for safe childbirth, trauma and H1N1 response (WHO, 2007).

A checklist is a "list of action items, tasks or behaviors arranged in a consistent manner, which allows the evaluator to record the presence or absence of the individual items listed" (Hales, Terblanche, Fowler, & Sibbald, 2007, p. 24). An effective checklist contains important criteria and limits extraneous or non-essential actions. Checklists can be in paper or electronic format and should be user-friendly within the work structure (Verdaasdonk, Stassen, Widhiasmara, & Dankelman, 2008).

Clinical checklists can take on several formats, depending on need and target process (Table 3.6). Using a tested checklist is optimal, but most published options are from traditional settings and require adaptation. Checklist design should consider the order of elements, layout of information, font size, and clarity of directions (Verdaasdonk et al., 2008). A sample of users should pilot the checklist to provide feedback for adjustment before full implementation.

Checklists improve safety in highly specialized and technical settings where repetitive functions can lead to complacency. Fragmented and chaotic care environments are filled with interruptions and distractions that can generate omissions of important steps in a clinical process. Checklists can be incorporated into correctional health care practice for high-risk processes. Below are some correctional health care processes that might benefit from use of a checklist.

- *Suicide Watch Release*: Steps to clear an inmate from suicide watch, including whom to notify and who needs to sign off on the release.

- *Chronic Care Visit Prep*: Necessary paperwork, specialty consults and diagnostic studies, and patient teaching materials.

- *Post-emergency Response*: List of necessary forms and documentation, restocking of medications and equipment, contact list and disposition of the patient.

- *Return from an Outside Appointment*: Medical record return, instructions from specialist, provider contact, and follow-up appointment scheduled for transport.

Eliminating Error-Prone Abbreviations

Written communications are an important component of clinical interaction. Whether handwritten or electronic, the medical record is a permanent record of communication among care providers as to the status and treatment of a patient.

Table 3.6. Types of Clinical Checklists

Type of Checklist	Description
Laundry list	Items, tasks or criteria are grouped into related categories with no particular order
Sequential or weakly sequential checklist	The grouping, order or overall flow of the items, tasks or criteria is relevant in order to obtain a valid outcome
Iterative checklist	Items, tasks or criteria on the checklist require repeated passes of review in order to obtain valid results, as early checkpoints may be altered by results entered in later checkpoints
Diagnostic checklist	Items, tasks or criteria on the checklist are formatted based on a "flowchart" model with the ultimate goal of drawing broad conclusions
Criteria of merit checklist (COM list)	The order, categorization and flow of information is paramount for the objectivity and reliability of the conclusions drawn; commonly used for evaluative purposes

Adapted from Hales et al., 2007

Abbreviations and shorthand can significantly increase chances of misinterpretation and clinical error. Correctional experts recommend reducing the use of abbreviations in communication about medical care (Stern et al., 2010). The Joint Commission (TJC) found that as much as 5% of communication errors concern the use of just a handful of misinterpreted abbreviations in medication orders (Brunetti, Santell, & Hicks, 2007). This finding led to the initiation of a 'Do Not Use' list of abbreviations for medication orders and other communication as part of their National Patient Safety Goals (Table 3.7). A surprising 43% of written errors were attributed to the use of 'QD' meaning 'once daily' (Brunetti, Santell, & Hicks, 2007). Eliminating this single abbreviation from clinical documentation significantly reduces communication error.

The Joint Commission "Do Not Use" list is a good start, but it was created in 2004 and has not been revised with new data. The Institute for Safe Medical Practices (ISMP) has a more extensive listing and includes abbreviations that TJC is

Table 3.7. TJC Do Not Use List of Abbreviations[1]

Do Not Use	Potential Problem	Use Instead
U, u (unit)	Mistaken for "0" (zero), the number "4" (four), or "cc"	Write "unit"
IU (International Unit)	Mistaken for IV (intravenous) or the number 10 (ten)	Write "International Unit"
Q.D., QD, q.d., qd (daily) Q.O.D., QOD, q.o.d., qod (every other day)	Mistaken for each other Periods after Q mistaken for "I" and the "O" mistaken for "I"	Write "daily" Write "every other day"
Trailing zero (X.0 mg)* Lack of leading zero (.X mg)	Decimal point is missing	Write "X mg" Write "0.X mg"
MS MSO$_4$ and MgSO$_4$	Can mean morphine sulfate or magnesium sulfate Confused for one another	Write "morphine sulfate" Write "magnesium sulfate"

[1]*Applies to all orders and all medication-related documentation that is handwritten (including free-text computer entry) or on pre-printed forms.*

*Exception: A 'trailing zero' may be used only where required to demonstrate the level of precision of the value being reported, such as for laboratory results, imaging studies that report size of lesions, or catheter/tube sizes. It may not be used in medication orders or other medication-related documentation.

© *The Joint Commission, 2014. Reprinted with permission*

considering for inclusion in the "Do Not Use" list. The following abbreviations have also been found to contribute to clinical error.

- The symbols ">" and "<"

- All abbreviations for drug names

- Apothecary Units

- The symbol "@"

- The abbreviation "cc"

- The abbreviation "Mg"

The use of symbols is also problematic in communication among multidisciplinary team members. Each discipline within a health care team can have a unique set of commonly understood symbols. Professionals in other disciplines, however, can easily misinterpret the meaning of symbols and abbreviations outside their field. One study found significant ambiguity and misinterpretation of symbol use among physicians and nurses from a variety of specialties (Galliers, Wilson, Randell, & Woodward, 2011). Standardizing – or avoiding – abbreviations in multidisciplinary communication is an important way to enhance safety.

Reading Back Verbal Orders

Verbal orders are another opportunity for communication error. Orders communicated verbally are common in all clinical settings, with estimates as high as 20% of all in-patient ordering (Wakefield & Wakefield, 2009). A verbal order is distinguished from other orders as being communicated orally by telephone, via digital device, or face-to-face. A nurse or other legally authorized individual transcribes the verbal order, and the prescriber later reviews and signs the transcribed order (Wakefield & Wakefield, 2009).

Errors reported in the literature concerning verbal orders include misinterpreting the number fifteen (15) as fifty (50) and the number two (2) as ten (10) and sound-alike medications. Examples cited include mistaking azithromycin for erythromycin and klonopin for clonidine (PA Patient Safety Authority, 2006). Verbal information among care providers can also be misinterpreted. Verbal communication of blood glucose readings without confirmation have resulted in administration of overdoses of insulin, as when the nurse heard a verbal report of the patient's blood glucose reading being 353 when the reading was actually reported as 85 (PA Patient Safety Authority, 2006).

For these reasons, correctional health care experts recommend a standing policy that all verbal orders be stated back (or read back) to the prescriber before implementation (Stern et al., 2010). This can include high-risk clinical information that results in medication administration such as blood glucose levels or patient assessment information during a code. One pediatric hospital reduced verbal order errors from 9% to zero by implementing this process (Doyle, 2006). The read-back process requires the staff member who receives a verbal order to read the order information aloud and obtain affirmation from the prescriber that the information is accurate. To reduce sound-alike errors in medication and dosage, the reader should spell out the medication name and dosage amount; for example, t-w-o – 2 mg.

The high risk of error with verbal orders requires limits on use. Wakefield and Wakefield (2009) provide some standard limits to verbal orders that should be considered in the correctional setting.

- Limit verbal orders to urgent patient care needs and not as a routine practice or for convenience purposes.

- Limit the staff who can take verbal orders.

- Limit the type of medication that can be ordered to formulary medications that are more likely to be familiar to all staff members.

- Do not use verbal orders for complex medication regimens such as chemotherapy.

Identification of the calling prescriber is also important. Health care staff can be surprisingly trusting when taking patient orders by phone, and correctional health professionals are no exception. One study found that few smaller institutions asked for identification when prescribers called with patient orders (Wakefield et al., 2012). With the rapid turnover of staff and covering providers, it can be risky to rely on voice recognition to confirm identification. Many large academic institutions use provider identification numbers for verbal orders. In several incidents individuals posing as providers have fooled staff into taking and implementing verbal orders for patients (ISMP, 2008). Methods should be in place to positively identify prescribers providing orders by telephone.

Structured Verbal Communication Frameworks

Verbal communication, especially in an urgent situation, can be muddied by too much information or hindered by too little. A structured communication framework speeds communication of important and necessary information and assists in critical decision-making in such high reliability industries as aviation and nuclear power. A physician coordinator of clinical informatics applied this concept to health care communication and created the SBAR communication format (Table 3.8) (O'Daniel & Rosenstein, 2008). When team members use the SBAR format to communicate a patient's condition, the speaker has a structure around which to organize the information, and the hearer has a framework for making decisions about the clinical information received.

The Joint Commission recommends structured communication such as SBAR for all patient hand-offs, including shift changes and discharges (Haig et al., 2006). The use of structured communication systems can improve communication during patient status changes and when responsibility for patient care is transferred to another provider (Rosenthal, 2013). The SBAR framework can be helpful for standard communication processes in correctional health care for situations such as these.

- Calling an off-site provider about a patient situation

- Handing-off infirmary patients at shift change

- Transferring patients to and from the emergency room, hospital or same-day surgical center

- Handing-off complex patients to family members at release

SBAR improves communication in a variety of clinical settings and among multiple disciplines (Haig et al., 2006). Using SBAR in one acute care setting showed significant reduction in unexpected deaths and increased unplanned admissions to intensive care (De Meester, Verspuy, Monsieurs, & Van Bogaert, 2013). Although there is no literature describing outcomes from the use of SBAR in the correctional setting, implementation of SBAR in a long-term care setting reported that the majority of nurses found the tool useful for organizing data and the majority of providers thought it improved communication about patient changes requiring action (Renz, Boltz, Wagner, Capezuti, & Lawrence, 2013). Correctional health care is similar to the long-term care environment in that both settings rely heavily on consultation with off-site providers who are often unfamiliar with the patient population, and both settings have a high percentage of LPN/LVN care givers. Because of these similarities, findings from use of communication tools in long-term care can be applied in correctional health care.

Patient Safety Huddles

Huddles are short, real-time team meetings to inform, anticipate needs, and make plans for short-term clinical needs (Manning, 2006). Structured questioning and brief updates enhance patient safety by alerting all team members to current particular concerns. In addition to being brief, these meetings should be held at the start of a shift and used to set mutual priorities for a functional work group (Dingley, Daugherty, Derieg, & Persing, 2008). Manning (2006) suggests the following questions to guide the discussion.

- What are the patient safety risks on the unit today?

- Is anyone worried or concerned about any particular patient?

- Do any patients need close observation that we all need to know about?

- Are there any new medications or equipment that might cause a safety risk?

- Identify and introduce new or re-assigned staff

Safety briefings may be challenging to introduce into the busy schedule of a clinical unit. Once in operation, however, staff often find that huddles provide for open communication among the various disciplines and prevent surprises about patient status (Nadzam, 2009). Stewart and Johnson (2007) successfully

Table 3.8. SBAR Structured Communication Model

Component	Description	Content Communicated
S-Situation	Briefly describe the patient-related issue	Identify speaker, location, and patient of concern Describe reason for call (if urgent, say so)
B-Background	Describe the clinical background of the situation, including pertinent patient history	Patient presenting complaint Relevant past medical history Brief summary of background
A-Assessment	State what you think the problem is	Relevant assessment findings, including vital signs and severity of condition Speaker's clinical impressions of the patient's status
R – Recommendation	Make a recommendation for correcting the problem	Speaker's suggestions of actions needed Speaker's explanation of what is required and how urgently

Adapted from Haig, Sutton, & Whittington, 2006

implemented huddles in an office setting and suggest strategies for success based on their experience.

- Get provider buy-in

- Set a consistent meeting time

- Experiment with different participants

- Limit sessions to 7 minutes or less

- Hold huddles in a central location

- Have everyone stand the entire time

- Designate a huddle leader

- Keep a standard agenda

- Designate a huddle champion

Bedside Hand-offs

Exchanging vital information across shifts can be particularly problematic in the correctional setting. The mix of ambulatory, emergency and sub-acute services can seem chaotic at the best of times. A structured process for shift hand-offs is a necessary part of safe patient communication. Loss of follow-through on important processes or patient status changes can result from gaps in communication among shifts.

A structured verbal process for shift hand-off improves patient safety by reducing the potential for lost information. Although many correctional settings rely on written information notebooks or audiotaped reports for shift report, these communication methods reduce accountability of off-going staff and do not allow on-coming staff to ask questions or clarify information (Laws & Amato, 2010). The move to a verbal hand-off seems like it would take extra time; however, studies indicate that this communication process has decreased overtime and improved the ability of nursing staff to respond to questions from providers early in the shift (Anderson & Mangino, 2006). A structured verbal hand-off process at shift change has promise for application in the correctional infirmary in conjunction with bedside rounding. In the ambulatory care section, communication of key conditions in the general population and emergency activities could take place using a verbal hand-off report.

Visualization – Whiteboards

Traditional whiteboards are a simple way of communicating important patient care information across various disciplines that may not have face-to-face contact. The low-tech, low-cost, and low-maintenance features of whiteboards make them ideal additions to communication efforts in the correctional setting. Whiteboards have been found to improve patient flow and discharge planning while establishing common knowledge of patient status in a clinic setting (Chaboyer, Wallen, Wallis, & McMurray, 2009). When used in patient rooms, whiteboards effectively involve patients in their care and facilitate frontline staff communication at the bedside (Sehgal, Green, Vidyarthi, Blegen, & Wachter, 2010). Whiteboards have many potential uses in the correctional setting. Boards in staff-only areas can be used to communicate patient status and process information (Table 3.9).

Whiteboards should be used with caution, especially related to patient confidentiality. Placement of the board should take access to the information into consideration. For example, whiteboards using patient names should be limited to locked staff areas. Responsibility for updating whiteboard information is also a concern. Communicating dated or incorrect information can be more harmful than no communication at all.

Table 3.9. Potential Uses of Whiteboards in Correctional Settings

Patient Information	Process Information
Those on alcohol or drug withdrawal requiring serial assessments	A laundry list of low stock medications for reorder
Those being released and needing medical/medication supplies	The location of staff members out in the compound and their expected return
Diabetics in the general population with special needs	Post-duty assignments such as who will respond to man-down emergencies on each shift
Highly allergic individuals with allergy and cell location	

Summary

Systems of therapeutic action are necessary in a highly chaotic and complex patient care system such as correctional health care. Standardizing tightly coupled processes in health care delivery can reduce opportunities for clinical error. High reliability organizational principles can apply to the correctional health care setting to guide practice. Methods for improving clinical systems include implementing human factor engineering concepts such as standardizing tasks, reducing the number of hand-offs, and improving information access while reducing reliance on memory. Improving teamwork and team communication contributes to a safe patient environment. Implementing structured communication processes such as checklists, verbal order read-back, structured verbal communication frameworks, huddles, bedside hand-offs, and whiteboards enhances and standardizes information sharing and reduces potential for error.

References

AHRQ. (2010). *TeamSTEPPS: Strategies & Tools to Enhance Performance and Patient Safety. Pocket Guide.* Washington, DC: Government Printing Office.

Anderson, C.D. & Mangino, R.R. (2006). Nurse shift report: who says you can't talk in front of the patient? *Nursing Administration Quarterly, 30* (2), 112–122.

American Organization of Nurse Executives (AONE). (2005). *AONE Guiding Principles for Excellence in Nurse-Physician Relationships.* American Organization of Nurse Executives. Retrieved from http://www.aone.org/resources/PDFs/AONE_GP_Excellence_Nurse_Physician.pdf

Arford, P.H. (2005). Nurse-physician communication: an organizational accountability. *Nursing Economic$, 23*(2), 72–77.

Baker, D.P., Gustafson, S., Beaubien, J.M., Salas, E., & Barach, P. (2005). Medical team training Programs in health care. In K. Henriksen, J. B. Battles, E. S. Marks, & D. I. Lewin (Eds.), *Advances in patient safety: From research to implementation (Volume 4: Programs, tools, and products).* Rockville, MD: Agency for Healthcare Research and Quality (US).

Barnsteiner, J.H. (2012). Safety. In G. Sherwood (Ed.), *Quality and safety in nursing: A competency approach to improving outcomes* (pp. 149–169). Chichester, West Sussex, UK: Wiley-Blackwell.

Brunetti, L., Santell, J.P., & Hicks, R.W. (2007). The impact of abbreviations on patient safety. *Joint Commission Journal on Quality and Patient Safety / Joint Commission Resources, 33*(9), 576–583.

Burke, C.S. (2004). How to turn a team of experts into an expert medical team: Guidance from the aviation and military communities. *Quality and Safety in Health Care, 13* (suppl_1), i96–i104. doi:10.1136/qshc.2004.009829

Carroll, J.S. & Rudolph, J.W. (2006). Design of high reliability organizations in health care. *Quality and Safety in Health Care, 15* (suppl_1), i4–i9. doi:10.1136/qshc.2005.015867

Chaboyer, W., Wallen, K., Wallis, M., & McMurray, A.M. (2009). Whiteboards: One tool to improve patient flow. *The Medical Journal of Australia, 190* (11 Suppl), S137–S140.

Coburn, A.F. & Gage-Croll, Z. (2011). Improving hospital patient safety through teamwork: The use of TeamSTEPPS in critical access hospitals. *Challenge, 5, 7.*

De Meester, K., Verspuy, M., Monsieurs, K.G., & Van Bogaert, P. (2013). SBAR improves nurse-physician communication and reduces unexpected death: A pre and post intervention study. *Resuscitation, 84*(9), 1192–1196. doi:10.1016/j.resuscitation.2013.03.016

Dekker, S. (2011). *Patient safety: A human factors approach.* Boca Raton, FL: CRC Press.

Dingley, C., Daugherty, K., Derieg, M.K., & Persing, R. (2008). Improving patient safety through provider communication strategy enhancements. In *Advances in patient safety: New directions and alternative approaches (Vol. 3:*

Performance and tools). Rockville, MD: Agency for Healthcare Research and Quality (US).

Disch, J. (2012). Teamwork and collaboration. In G. Sherwood & J. Barnsteiner (Ed.), Quality and safety in nursing: *A competency approach to improving outcomes* (pp. 91–112). Ames, IA: Wiley-Blackwell.

Doyle, E. (2006). To prevent ordering errors, one hospital is bringing "read back" to the bedside. *Today's Hospitalist*. Retrieved from http://todayshospitalist. com/index.php?b=articles_read&cnt=106

Elderkin-Thompson, V. & Waitzkin, H. (1999). Differences in clinical communication by gender. *Journal of General Internal Medicine*, 14(2), 112–121. doi:10.1046/j.1525-1497.1999.00296.x

Emanuel, L., Berwick, D., Conway, J., Combes, J., Hatlie, M., Leape, L., … Walton, M. (2008). What exactly is patient safety? *Advances in Patient Safety: New Directions and Alternative Approaches, 1*. Retrieved from http://ahrq.hhs. gov/downloads/pub/ advances2/vol1/Advances-Emanuel-Berwick_110.pdf

Fagan, M.J. (2012). Techniques to improve patient safety in hospitals. *JONA: The Journal of Nursing Administration*, 42(9), 426–430. doi:10.1097/NNA.0b013e3182664df5

Ferguson, S.,L. (2008). TeamSTEPPS: Integrating teamwork principles into adult health/medical-surgical practice. *MEDSURG Nursing*, 17(2), 122–125.

Fewster-Thuente, L. & Velsor-Friedrich, B. (2008). Interdisciplinary collaboration for healthcare professionals. *Nursing Administration Quarterly*, 32(1), 40–48.

Galliers, J., Wilson, S., Randell, R., & Woodward, P. (2011). Safe use of symbols in handover documentation for medical teams. *Behaviour & Information Technology*, 30(4), 499–506. doi:10.1080/0144929X.2011.582147

Gosbee, J. (2002). Human factors engineering and patient safety. *Quality and Safety in Health Care*, 11(4), 352–354.

Graham, K.C. & Cvach, M. (2010). Monitor alarm fatigue: Standardizing use of physiological monitors and decreasing nuisance alarms. *American Journal of Critical Care, 19*(1), 28–34. doi:10.4037/ajcc2010651

Haig, K.M., Sutton, S., & Whittington, J. (2006). SBAR: A shared mental model for improving communication between clinicians. *Joint Commission Journal on Quality and Patient Safety, 32*(3), 167–175.

Hales, B., Terblanche, M., Fowler, R., & Sibbald, W. (2007). Development of medical checklists for improved quality of patient care. *International Journal for Quality in Health Care, 20*(1), 22–30. doi:10.1093/intqhc/mzm062

Healthcare Risk Management. (2012). Hospital cuts med errors 30%, falls 88% with TeamSTEPPS. *Healthcare Risk Management, 34*(8), 90.

Hines, S., Luna, K., Loftus, J., Marquardt, M., & Stelmokas, D. (2008). *Becoming a high reliability organization: Operational advice for hospital leaders*. Rockville, MD: Agency for Healthcare Research and Quality.

Institute for Safe Medication Practices (ISMP). (2008). Telephone orders: Do you know the caller is for real? *ISMP Nurse Advise-ERR, 6*(7), 2.

Interprofessional Education Collaborative Expert Panel. (2011). *Core competencies for interprofessional collaborative practice: Report of an expert panel.* Washington, DC: Interprofessional Education Collaborative.

Klejka, D.E. (2012). Shhh! Conducting a quiet zone pilot study for medication safety. *Nursing, 42*(9), 18–21. doi:10.1097/01.NURSE.0000418623.06842.59

Laws, D. & Amato, S. (2010). Incorporating bedside reporting into change-of-shift report. *Rehabilitation Nursing, 35*(2), 70–74.

Manning, M.L. (2006). Improving clinical communication through structured conversation. *Nursing Economic$, 24*(5), 268–271.

Manser, T. (2009). Teamwork and patient safety in dynamic domains of healthcare: A review of the literature. *Acta Anaesthesiologica Scandinavica, 53*(2), 143–151. doi:10.1111/j.1399-6576.2008.01717.x

Maxwell, D., Grenny, J., McMillan, R., Patterson, K., & Switzler, A. (2005). Silence kills: *The seven crucial conversations in healthcare.* Retrieved from www.aacn.org/WD/Practice/Docs/PublicPolicy/SilenceKills.pdf

McKeon, L.M., Oswaks, J.D., & Cunningham, P.D. (2006). Safeguarding patients: Complexity science, high reliability organizations, and implications for team training in healthcare. *Clinical Nurse Specialist, 20*(6), 298–304.

Murray, J.S. (2009). Workplace bullying in nursing: a problem that can't be ignored. *MedSurg Nursing, 18*(5), 273–276.

Nadzam, D.M. (2009). Nurses' role in communication and patient safety. *Journal of Nursing Care Quality, 24*(3), 184–188.

O'Daniel, M. & Rosenstein, A.H. (2008). Professional communication and team collaboration. *Patient Safety and Quality: An Evidence-Based Handbook for Nurses, 2,* 08–0043.

PA Patient Safety Authority. (2006). Improving the safety of telephone or verbal orders. *PA-PSRS Patient Safety Advisory, 3*(2), 1–5.

Petri, L. (2010). Concept analysis of interdisciplinary collaboration. *Nursing Forum, 45*(2), 73–82.

Reason, J. (2000). Human error: Models and management. *BMJ: British Medical Journal, 320*(7237), 768.

Renz, S.M., Boltz, M.P., Wagner, L.M., Capezuti, E.A., & Lawrence, T.E. (2013). Examining the feasibility and utility of an SBAR protocol in long-term care. *Geriatric Nursing, 34*(4), 295–301. doi:10.1016/j.gerinurse.2013.04.010

Riser, D.T., Simon, R., Rice, M.M., Salisbury, M.L., & Morey, J.C. (2011). A structured teamwork system to reduce clinical errors. In P. Spath (Ed.), *Error reduction in health care: A systems approach to improving patient safety* (pp. 297–334). San Francisco, CA: Jossey-Bass.

Rivera, A.J. & Karsh, B.T. (2010). Interruptions and distractions in healthcare: Review and reappraisal. *Quality & Safety in Health Care, 19*(4), 304–312. doi:10.1136/qshc.2009.033282

Roberts, K. H., & Rousseau, D. M. (1989). Research in nearly failure-free, high-reliability organizations: Having the bubble. *IEEE Transactions on Engineering Management, 36*(2), 132-139.

Rosenthal, L. (2013). Enhancing communication between night shift RNs and hospitalists: An opportunity for performance improvement. *JONA: The Journal of Nursing Administration, 43*(2), 59–61. doi:10.1097/NNA.0b013e31827f200b

Sayre, M.M., McNeese-Smith, D., Leach, L.S., & Phillips, L.R. (2012). An educational intervention to increase "speaking-up" behaviors in nurses and improve patient safety. *Journal of Nursing Care Quality, 27*(2), 154–160. doi:10.1097/NCQ.0b013e318241d9ff

Sehgal, N.L., Green, A., Vidyarthi, A.R., Blegen, M.A., & Wachter, R.M. (2010). Patient whiteboards as a communication tool in the hospital setting: A survey of practices and recommendations. *Journal of Hospital Medicine, 5*(4), 234–239. doi:10.1002/jhm.638

Selle, K.M., Salamon, K., Boarman, R., & Sauer, J. (2008). Providing interprofessional learning through interdisciplinary collaboration: The role of "modelling." *Journal of Interprofessional Care, 22*(1), 85–92. doi:10.1080/13561820701714755

Semel, M.E., Resch, S., Haynes, A.B., Funk, L.M., Bader, A., Berry, W.R., ... Gawande, A.A. (2010). Adopting a surgical safety checklist could save money and improve the quality of care in U.S. hospitals. *Health Affairs, 29*(9), 1593–1599. doi:10.1377/hlthaff.2009.0709

Shekelle, P.G., Pronovost, P.J., Wachter, R.M., McDonald, K.M., Schoelles, K., Dy, S.M., ... Angood, P.B. (2013). The top patient safety strategies that can be encouraged for adoption now. *Annals of Internal Medicine, 158*(5), 365–368.

Spath, P. (2011). *Error reduction in health care: A systems approach to improving patient safety.* San Francisco, CA: Jossey-Bass.

Sportsman, S. & Hamilton, P. (2007). Conflict management styles in nursing and allied health professionals. *Journal of Professional Nursing, 23*(3), 157–166.

Stern, M.F., Greifinger, R.B., & Mellow, J. (2010). Patient safety: Moving the bar in prison health care standards. *American Journal of Public Health, 100*(11), 2103.

Stewart, E.E. & Johnson, B.C. (2007). Huddles: Improve office efficiency in mere minutes. *Family Practice Management.* Retrieved from www.aafp.org/fpm/2007/0600/p27.pdf

The Joint Commission (TJC). (2013) *Root causes by event type* 2004-2013. Retrieved from www.jointcommission.org/assets/1/18/Root_Causes_by_Event_Type_2004-2Q2013.pdf

Verdaasdonk, E.G., Stassen, L.P., Widhiasmara, P.P., & Dankelman, J. (2008). Requirements for the design and implementation of checklists for surgical processes. *Surgical Endoscopy, 23*(4), 715–726. doi:10.1007/s00464-008-0044-4

Wachter, R.M. (2012). *Understanding patient safety.* New York, NY: McGraw Hill Medical.

Wakefield, D.S. & Wakefield, B.J. (2009). Are verbal orders a threat to patient safety? *Postgraduate Medical Journal, 85*(1007), 460–463. doi:10.1136/qshc.2009.034041

Wakefield, D.S., Wakefield, B.J., Despins, L., Brandt, J., Davis, W., Clements, K., & Steinmann, W. (2012). A review of verbal order policies in acute care hospitals. *Joint Commission Journal on Quality and Patient Safety, 38*(1), 24–33.

Woods, M.S. (2006). How communication complicates the patient safety movement. *Patient Safety & Quality Healthcare*. Retrieved from www.psqh.com/mayjun06/dun.html

World Health Organization (WHO). (2007). *Communication During Patient Hand-Overs, 1*(3), 4. Retrieved from http://www.who.int/patientsafety/solutions/patientsafety/PS-Solution3.pdf

Xyrichis, A. & Ream, E. (2008). Teamwork: A concept analysis. *Journal of Advanced Nursing, 61*(2), 232–241. doi:10.1111/j.1365-2648.2007.04496.x

4 The Recipient of Care

As the recipient of care, the patient is a primary component of the patient safety system (Figure 4.1). The patient is more than a passive recipient of the care delivered by health care professionals. In a patient safety culture, engaging the patient as both the focus of care and an active team member goes a long way in reducing clinical error.

As a domain of patient safety (Table 4.1), the patient is the center of care provision around which all other activities revolve. Engagement of the patient in care delivery has challenges that must be overcome in the correctional setting.

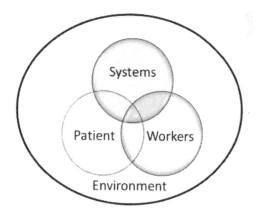

Figure 4.1 A Patient Safety Model of Health Care

Adapted from Emanuel et al., 2008

Patient-Centered Care

The concept of patient-centered care was originally described in *Crossing the Quality Chasm,* the Institute of Medicine (IOM) report on health care quality as "providing care that is respective of and responsive to individual patient preferences, needs, and values and ensuring that patient values guide all clinical decision" (IOM, 2001, p. 40). This is a difficult proposition in a secure environment where health care is not a primary goal, and is predominantly provider-centered and episodic in nature. Correctional patients are generally not trusted to be a part of the health care team - and certainly not the center of it. Yet the principles of patient-centered care, when applied in this setting, have opportunity to greatly decrease clinical error and increase compliance with the treatment plan.

Many traditional settings have expanded patient-centered care to be family-centered care, involving the values and concerns of family members in care decisions. This is particularly helpful for maternal-child health issues. Family involvement is difficult in the correctional setting because the security perimeter does not allow for direct contact and because many patients have estranged families.

Table 4.1 Domains and Principles of Patient Safety

Domain of Patient Safety	Principle of Patient Safety
Environment of Care	A Just Culture in a Learning Organization
Systems for Therapeutic Action	High Reliability System Design Communication and Teamwork
Recipient of Care	Patient-Centered Care
Health Care Workers	Competent Care Providers

Family members may be separated by great distances, as in the case of federal and state prison systems, or those housed in different states in rental beds.

The Institute for Patient- and Family-Centered Care's (IPFCC; n.d.) four core concepts of patient-centered practice provide a framework to discuss applying patient-centered care principles in the correctional setting (Table 4.2). Although the

Table 4.2. Core Concepts of Patient-Centered Care

Core Concept	Description
Dignity and Respect	Listening to and honoring the patient's and family's perspective. Considering the patient's knowledge, values, beliefs and cultural background in care decisions
Information Sharing	Sharing complete and unbiased information with patients and families
Participation	Encouraging and supporting the patient's involvement in health care
Collaboration	Collaborating with patients and families about policy and program development, facility design and professional education

Adapted from IPFCC, n.d.

limiting nature of the patient relationship in corrections prohibits full implementation, practical application of most patient-centered care concepts is indeed possible and advantageous to patient safety and risk reduction.

Dignity and Respect

Patient-centered care values the patient's and family's perspective about health care. The patient's understanding of the importance of the condition and past experiences in the health care system often influence the description of symptoms. The incarcerated patient can also bring maladaptive communication patterns and value manipulation over honest discussion, further clouding communication. Listening to and honoring the patient, at the level of involvement they are capable of, can reveal the true symptoms under investigation and lead to a quicker, more accurate diagnosis.

Information Sharing

During incarceration, inmates have little to no control over the day-to-day decisions that directly affect them. They have limited food choices, exercise is timed, and they are required to follow an established schedule for everything from when they shower to when they have their meals. In contrast, a major principle of health care ethics is patient autonomy in health care decisions. Fully sharing information about disease process and informed decision-making allow some aspects of self-determination in the health care relationship. Full information sharing also assists in patient safety, as an informed patient is more likely to continue in therapy and develop healthy self-care practices (Spath, 2004).

Participation

Patient-centered care requires the patient's active participation in the program of care. Information sharing supports patient participation, as does the structure of care delivery. This means, where possible, having the patient develop self-care skills such as taking blood glucose readings and blood pressure checks. When security limitations make this impossible, verbally guide the patient through the steps to perform a health care function, and ascertain understanding. This will help the patient continue to care for themselves on re-entry to society.

Collaboration

Collaborating over policy, procedure, and design of health care is probably the patient-centered care principle least able to be implemented in a correctional setting. Soliciting patient input into such decisions, however, may have surprising benefits. Some institutions have inmate councils for airing general concerns. These meetings may be used to discuss health care processes to gain insight and support. For example, inmates may have valuable perspectives to share about the sick call process or medication administration in the housing area. If a process is not functioning smoothly, particularly one that requires inmate initiation or action, collaboration with selected inmates may reveal misconceptions and may generate ideas for revisions to improve use and application.

Possibly one of the most practical goals of patient-centered care comes from Epstein, Fiscella, Lesser, and Strange (2010) as "providing the right care for the right person at the right time" (p. 2). By focusing on these "rights", correctional health care providers center on the patient rather than on the disease, care provider, technology, or organization. This is a helpful goal in an organizational structure such as the criminal justice system, where patient preferences, needs, and values are not often a primary concern.

Patient-centered care is the right thing to do on moral and ethical grounds, but it is also the right thing to do from a patient safety perspective. This care model has been shown to improve patient outcomes and reduce care costs (Epstein et al., 2010; Weiner et al., 2013).

> "One case I recalled very well was a patient who was refusing his insulin for diabetes. We called his mom and spoke with her about ways we might convince him to comply with treatment. Eventually, we were successful when we brought him to a room where we could call her directly and have her talk to him. Even though he was an adult and in his 40's or 50's, men never stop listening to their mothers."
> – Kathy Wild, Correctional Healthcare Consultant and Former Deputy Agency Director for Correctional Health Services at the Orange County Heath Care Agency in Santa Ana, CA

The Role of Patients in Individual Safety

In addition to being the center of care, patients have a role to play in maintaining patient safety. Encouraging patient involvement is an important aspect of correctional health care delivery because it prepares patients for self-care upon re-entry into society. This involvement has an added benefit of providing another mechanism of error reduction. Correctional health care providers should also consider family involvement as a component of patient safety.

Vincent and Coulter (2002) identify six basic areas of patient involvement in care that promote safety.

- Choosing a suitable provider

- Assisting in reaching an accurate diagnosis

- Providing input into an appropriate treatment plan

- Monitoring treatment administration

- Identifying side effects and adverse effects of treatment

- Involving family and friends, whenever able

At least five of these six areas apply in the correctional setting. The ability to choose a care provider (the first recommendation) is limited while incarcerated; however, patients can be encouraged to be involved in reaching an accurate diagnosis, coming up with a treatment plan that will work within the limitations of the correctional setting, monitoring the administration of the prescribed treatment, and identifying side effects or adverse effects of the treatment regimen.

Even in the correctional environment, involvement of family and friends can elicit greater patient safety. Family members can provide needed history on past treatment and medication regimens. They can provide contact information for various health care providers and confirm responses to treatments that the patient has had.

Reaching an Accurate Diagnosis

An accurate diagnosis requires an open and honest dialogue between patient and care provider. Patients must sometimes share uncomfortable information. A sympathetic and listening approach is necessary. Without full information exchange, diagnostic errors can result (Vincent & Coulter, 2002). Yet health care providers must also balance potential manipulation or secondary gain issues in the correctional setting. Further, as a purveyor of privileges in the prison culture, sympathetic health care staff can be seen as an easy "mark" for obtaining beneficial perks such as lower bunks, special shoes, or limited work duty (Paris, 2006).

Treatment Plan Input

The patient's input into the treatment plan may assist with effectiveness, especially in planning treatment that might have adherence or motivational issues. While specific medication choices for the condition might not be in a patient's purview, shared decision-making when equally effective options are available may result in better outcomes. For example, medication adherence may improve with once-a-day dosing rather than three-times-daily dosing. Fully understanding the patient's living restrictions can also affect treatment planning. Restricted living space and limited financial resources affect activity choices and commissary purchases. Active patient involvement in initial treatment planning can overcome obstacles.

Treatment Monitoring

A major role for patients in improving safe outcomes is monitoring the treatment plan and questioning actions or components that they do not understand. This most often takes place at the point of care delivery and can include questioning new medications or even asking if the provider has washed his or her hands (Holme, 2009). Depending on a patient's personality and background, questioning an authority may be difficult. Some patients may need encouragement to act as their

Table 4.3. Speak-Up Patient Involvement Actions

Letter	Description
S	Speak up if you have questions or concerns. If you still don't understand, ask again. It's your body and you have a right to know.
P	Pay attention to the care you get. Always make sure you're getting the right treatments and medicines by the right health care professionals. Don't assume anything.
E	Educate yourself about your illness. Learn about the medical tests you get and your treatment plan.
A	Ask a trusted family member or friend to be your advocate (advisor or supporter).
K	Know what medicines you take and why you take them. Medicine errors are the most common health care mistakes.
U*	Use a hospital, clinic, surgery center or other type of health care organization that has been carefully checked out. For example, TJC visits hospitals to see if they are meeting its quality standards.
P	Participate in all decisions about your treatment. You are the center of the health care team.

Adapted from TJC Facts about Speak-Up, 2013

*not possible in the correctional setting

own patient safety advocates. The Joint Commission's Speak-Up patient safety campaign provides encouragement for patient involvement in error reduction (Table 4.3). With the exception of one, these action categories have application in the correctional setting.

Although patients can, and should, participate in their own safety, the primary responsibility for patient safety remains with care providers. That being acknowledged, a first step in involving patients in their own health care safety is to inform them of their role. This can take place at initial screening or at a first clinic visit. Patients should know that providers expect them to be an active participant in their care and that they need to engage health care staff when they have questions about a diagnosis, treatment, or medication.

Identifying Side Effects and Adverse Effects of Treatment

A fully informed patient can also foster patient safety by being alert to side effects and adverse effects of the treatment plan. Practitioners should regularly engage patients in self-evaluation of any untoward effects of treatment and continually encourage patients to mention these, if present, to their care providers. Sick call protocols should always include patient instruction on what signs and symptoms indicate a need to contact a care provider. Some correctional health care staff may be unwilling to share information about potential side effects with patients for fear that this will be used to manipulate treatment. A better practice is to engage the patient in earnest dialogue about symptoms experienced and objectively evaluate the reported side effects.

> "With our terminal patients and some of our complex mental health clients, we involved the family to assist with decisions, know what we were doing with the courts, and help with follow-up after jail. In jails, it is difficult to involve the families, but it is worth it as it educates the families, helps them participate in their care and know what we are doing in jail and not leaving their loved ones without care and treatment... many, many benefits to involving families in complex cases and those refusing care."
>
> **– Gayle Burrow, Correctional Healthcare Consultant and Former Director of Corrections Health, Multnomah County Health Department, Portland, OR**

Family Participation

Although the security perimeter seems a barrier to active family involvement, distance communication methods (particularly telephone) can be used to engage willing family members to enhance patient safety. This can be particularly helpful if the patient is developmentally delayed or mentally ill. The following are suggestions for family involvement in correctional health care.

- Use a positive family relationship to motivate a patient to participate in the care plan.

- Obtain missing family and health history information necessary for the development of an effective treatment plan.

- Gain access to prior health records and provider contact information.

- Assist in continuity of care after incarceration.

Barriers to Patient Involvement

The many barriers to patient involvement in the correctional setting center on the care environment and the patient profile. An organizational evaluation of barriers to patient involvement is an important first step when seeking to engage patients to actively participate in their care and safety.

Paternal Organizational Culture

An organizational culture that devalues the patient and discourages patient input in other areas of practice will hinder patient involvement efforts. If a correctional culture is based on order, control, and discipline it could stall efforts to actively engage patients in care decisions and therapy monitoring. A paternalistic culture can develop in a correctional setting where inmates are controlled and are not expected to make personal decisions. This hinders patient engagement in their health care and reduces motivation toward self-care activities.

Lack of Patient Preparation

The patient population can be ill-prepared to actively participate in their own health care. Limited English proficiency and low basic literacy and health literacy levels can weaken engagement in treatment (Wachter, 2012). The inmate population is less educated than the general population and is twice as likely to have learning disabilities (Greenberg, Dunleavy, & Kutner, 2007). It is also difficult to get an accurate evaluation of literacy from the patient's self-report because inmates are more likely to over-estimate their reading and comprehension abilities (Amodeo, Jin, & Kling, 2009).

Patients' unwillingness to participate in their own care can also be a barrier. Negative prior experiences with the health care system -- prior medical errors, feeling rejected, being challenged to obtain health care, confrontational behavioral styles and the like -- can limit patient involvement, as can anticipation of negative responses from some in the health care team (Peat et al., 2010). Sometimes, patients are fearful of what will happen to them.

Practitioner Behaviors

Patients' involvement in their own care is affected by their willingness, knowledge and past experiences in the health care system (Spath, 2004). Likewise, practitioner behaviors can also inhibit patient involvement. Engaging patients in care provision involves a time commitment that clinicians may be unwilling or unable to make. In addition, a continuing paternalistic medical culture combined with pervasive attitudes about the correctional patient population can result in an authoritarian stance toward the patient that inhibits involvement. Pelling (2004) identified these practitioner behaviors that discourage open communication, and, therefore, patient involvement in their care and safety:

- Defending an action and blocking continued expression of concern
- Interrupting and finishing sentences for the patient
- Deliberately changing the subject when uncomfortable
- Citing policy as a reason for an action
- Minimizing patient's concerns
- Condescending comments about patient concerns
- Not following through on promises

Legal Liability

Another barrier to involving patients in safety activities is the perception that this may increase legal liability. Indeed, medical professionals are loath to indicate that errors happen in health care delivery, although most patients are aware of this fact. A culture of silence, however, has not been found helpful in persuading juries. In one nationwide study, jurors expected disclosure of clinical errors and perceived non-disclosure as cover-up and "hiding" responsibility (Saxton & Finkelstein, 2004). In an oft-quoted classic study of families initiating prenatal professional liability suits, the majority of families believed that physicians would not listen to them, would not talk openly about the error or were attempting to mislead them (Hickson, Clayton, Githens, & Sloan, 1992).

An apology can be a natural human response to error, but statements acknowledging error have been traditionally avoided in medical practice. Indeed, risk managers and legal counsel have advised against apology as it can be construed as an admission of guilt. Apologies in medical error situations, however, can decrease blame and anger while increasing trust and improve relationships (Robbennolt, 2009). Therefore, efforts are underway to revise both federal and state rules of evidence to exclude apologies as general admissions of fault (Pearlmutter, 2011).

The litigious patient population in the correctional setting gives health care providers pause to involve them in activities meant to improve patient safety; however, clearly, an open attitude toward the potential for clinical error is more advantageous in reducing litigation than defensiveness or silence.

Perceived Negative Effect

A final barrier to involving patients in promoting their own safety is the perceived negative effects to the patient. Depending on the patient's personal characteristics, this involvement could place an undue stress on an already disadvantaged situation (Entwistle, Mello, & Brennan, 2005). Very sick patients, in particular, may be unable to cope with responsibility for monitoring their own health care. Patients may also feel uncomfortable checking on and challenging actions of health care providers who may be deemed learned authority figures. Patients may worry that initiating a discussion about a possible error might label them as a troublemaker or affect what care they will have access to in the correctional setting.

Patient as Team Member

There are several key ways to involve the patient as a team member to improve patient safety in the larger health care delivery system. A literature review by Peat et al. (2010) found three areas of patient involvement in the traditional setting: informing the management plan, monitoring treatment delivery, and informing system improvements. These areas may also be appropriate in the correctional setting.

Informing the Management Plan

As identified earlier, the patient is an active part of the management plan, although they may not realize it without prompting. Patients can volunteer information from their past history that is vital to care decisions. Providers can elicit information by asking key questions about allergies and adverse reactions. Health care staff can encourage the patient to provide all possible information and then determine which information is relevant to the presenting condition.

Patients may also need encouragement to be forthright about the acceptability of a proposed treatment plan. The care provider in a correctional setting may not fully understand security restrictions and personal freedom limitations that affect the patient's ability to comply with the proposed plan.

Monitoring and Ensuring Safe Delivery of Treatment

The patient has several methods for monitoring and ensuring safe delivery of treatment. First, the patient is a check on treatment delivery by health care staff. For example, a practitioner may change a patient's hypertension medication during a chronic care visit. If the patient receives the old medication during the next medication line, the patient should ask about the medication, referencing the recent chronic care visit, and ask if the new medication has been received. Productive patient monitoring requires a team atmosphere in care delivery and open-mindedness among all staff members. Defensiveness about, or derision of, patient monitoring of treatment delivery will not encourage a safe patient culture.

Ensuring safe treatment delivery also involves treatment that is self-administered. Although less prevalent in the correctional setting than in the community due to security constraints, patients may self-administer keep-on-person (KOP) medications and simple wound treatments. Engaging the patient in safe care delivery, therefore, also involves thorough patient teaching and answering any remaining questions about their role in self-care.

Incarcerated patients can also participate in monitoring the completion and follow-through on diagnostic tests. Patients can be instructed to expect results of any diagnostic test performed, whether positive or negative. If the patient hears nothing about test results in a given time period, they can initiate a service request, thus prompting staff about the test and monitoring any processing or communication issues.

Informing System Improvements

Correctional health care staff may not initially see an opportunity for inmates to be a team member in system improvements; however, there can be surprising benefit from eliciting constructive feedback from this population. Patients prompt system improvements in traditional settings by providing individual feedback on current processes, acting as a patient representative on various committees and teams, and pilot-testing new interventions (Peat et al., 2010). Correctional settings can apply these principles, as well, through these actions.

- Engaging with current inmate involvement structures such as housing unit forums or inmate activity groups for feedback on current or proposed systems of care.

- Designating several cooperative and motivated inmates to be patient representatives to the health care unit.

- Having patients review or pilot new patient education materials.

- Asking for patient feedback on a new system of care delivery.

- Involving patients in improving situations such as refusals to come to clinic or declining to take medications.

- Using inmate health care grievances as an opportunity for system improvement.

Specific Practices to Promote Patient Involvement

Involving patients in their care, so as to improve patient safety, takes effort. Both staff and patient team members must develop skills to accomplish this. Patient engagement needs to become a normal and automatic part of the patient care process. Several specific patient involvement practices help create patient engagement in traditional health care settings, and applying these in the correctional setting can lead to reduced clinical error and improved patient safety.

Helping Patients Understand Their Role

Most patients, particularly those in the correctional setting, need help to understand their role in the patient care process. Attention to describing how health care is provided in the correctional setting, as well as the patient's role in obtaining care and maintaining health, should start at the point of entry into the system and continue throughout incarceration. Entry into a jail or prison can be overwhelming, and information overload can quickly ensue. Limiting early information to the process for contacting the medical unit for urgent and emergency care is a good place to start. Care providers can then build upon this foundation in later encounters at the initial physical assessment, sick call visits, and chronic care clinic appointments.

Because inmates can be quickly institutionalized into a passive role, it is important to clearly identify that health care staff expect them to take an active part in their health program. Spath (2004) suggests the following directions to patients that are applicable in a correctional setting. These guidelines can be incorporated into information and presentations about health care access.

- Be forthright with past medical and mental health history.

- Inform health care staff of current medications and allergies.

- Ask for an explanation of any unfamiliar medication or treatment.

- Ask for an explanation of any test or procedure that is ordered.

- Ask for test results and what they mean.

- Ask for clarification of schedules and forms.

Both patients and health care practitioners can be uncomfortable having patients address staff safety practices; however, this is becoming more prevalent in traditional settings and bears consideration in the correctional setting (Spath, 2004). Many settings encourage patients to question staff about the following practices, if there is concern.

- Hand washing if not viewed by the patient.

- Verifying identity if the staff member does not specifically ask the patient's name.

- Monitoring cleanliness of the health care area.

- Identifying clutter, water or uneven floor surfaces that might lead to slips or falls.

Improving Health Literacy

Health literacy, the ability of an individual to adequately understand basic health information and services, is needed to make appropriate health decisions (Nielsen-Bohlman, Panzer, & Kindig, 2004). Low health literacy affects patient safety by reducing chances of obtaining an accurate medical history, eliciting treatment adherence, and avoiding medication errors (Nielsen-Bohlman et al., 2004). Improving the health literacy of correctional patients reduces the risk of clinical error during incarceration and improves health outcomes after re-entry into society.

This complex group of skills moves far beyond merely the ability to read. For example, health literacy involves the ability to understand the implications of appointments, self-administration of medication and monitoring of symptoms, patient teaching materials, and consent forms. Health literacy is affected by belief systems and communication styles; therefore, culture can play a significant role in health literacy. It is also affected by education and language (Nielsen-Bohlman et al., 2004).

Several patient populations are particularly vulnerable to low health literacy. The elderly, minority and immigrant populations, and low-income adults score lower in basic health literacy skills than the general population. Intuitively, it is expected that learning disability or lower education level equates to lower health literacy levels, but even those from higher educational levels can have weak health literacy skills (Weiss, 2007).

There is little research into the health literacy of the correctional patient population, although all indications are that it is low. First, basic literacy among those in prison is lower than the general population (Amodeo et al., 2009); add to this the disproportionate percentage of low-income minority or immigrant adults in the prison population – all factors for lower health literacy among the general patient population. One of the few studies into health literacy factors in our patient population found that, of 358 adult male inmates in the Kentucky prison system, 27% had limited health literacy (Miller, Chung, Connell, Lennie, & Moser, 2012).

Health literacy and informed consent or refusal. A patient's understanding and application of health information is of particular importance during informed consent or refusal processes. Legal liability is high in these instances, yet a wealth of research indicates that most consent forms are written at a level beyond the health literacy level of the patient population (Nielsen-Bohlman et al., 2004). These high-risk documents should be examined first in the process of addressing patient safety by improving patient education materials.

Clues that a patient may have low health literacy. Some patients are embarrassed about low literacy and will not readily admit to needing help. Others may not even be aware of deficiency in health knowledge and skill. The following behaviors may be a clue that a patient is having trouble understanding health care information or instructions (Cornett, 2009).

- Making an excuse when asked to read or fill out paperwork such as "I don't have my glasses."
- Checking "no" on a health history to avoid follow-up questions.
- Missing appointments or making errors in medication dosing.
- Irritability, nervousness, confusion, or indifference during health care encounters.
- Identifying medications by color, size, or shape rather than name and purpose.
- Following directions literally.
- Holding written material closer to read, lack of visual focus on reading material, using a finger to point at the words.

When any of these behaviors are displayed, low health literacy should be considered and the approach adjusted to improve understanding.

Provide easy-to-understand written materials. Extensive studies confirm that most patient medical information materials are beyond average adult reading levels (Nielsen-Bohlman et al., 2004). A concrete step toward improving health literacy is to improve the readability of any patient handout used in health care delivery. Clear and understandable patient education materials for low-literacy audiences should be engaging, including graphics and pictures to demonstrate important principles (HHS, 2009). Materials should be limited to need-to-know information that directly tells the audience what they need to do using action terms. The writing style for information materials should be positive, friendly and conversational, using simple words with limited use of medical and scientific jargon. Statistics should be limited and use general terms such as "many" or "few". The format of the teaching material can also affect understanding. Font size of text should be as large as possible to improve readability, with a common recommendation of at least 12-point font size (HHS, 2009).

Once materials are written and formatted, readability should be tested. The best test is to pilot with a patient sampling; however, MS Word functions and online services can also factor readability. A very simple test of readability is the number of multiple-syllable words in the document. The Simple Measure of Gobbledygook (SMOG), developed and extensively tested in the 1960's, involves counting the multiple-syllable words in three strings of ten sentences within the document and then comparing the count to a table to determine reading level (McLaughlin, 1969).

Teach-back/demonstrate-back. Written materials are not the only incomprehensible communication in health care. Verbal communication is also often filled with complicated information that is difficult to digest. Care providers cannot rely on a patient's simple nod or affirmation that there are no questions as confirmation of understanding. Instead, providers should institute a teach-back or demonstrate-back process for all health care interactions where the patient must then use the information to make health care decisions, self-medicate, perform a treatment, or determine if symptoms warrant return to the health unit.

The teach-back concept involves asking the patient to verbally repeat back the information shared during a health care encounter to confirm an accurate understanding (Weiss, 2007). A modification of the process is to have the patient demonstrate the new health skill such as self-injection or dressing change. Consistent application of the teach-back process in patient teaching has been found to reduce readmissions (White, Garbez, Carroll, Brinker, & Howie-Esquivel, 2013) and improve comprehension of informed consent and privacy issues (Kripalani, Bengtzen, Henderson, & Jacobson, 2008).

Evaluation of the teach-back process in non-correctional health care settings indicates that staff must be taught the four key steps in order to be effective (Table 4.4). It is important, during the teach-back process, to use open-ended questions to initiate patient response; for example, ask the patient to describe how they will share what they learned with a friend or family member. Be sure they respond with all critical information.

Table 4.4. Steps of the Teach-Back Process

Step	Action
1	Explain the concept and/or demonstrate the skill
2	Ask the patient to explain the concept or demonstrate the skill
3	Identify and correct any misunderstanding or missed information or skill steps
4	Ask again for an explanation of the concept or demonstration of the skill
5	Repeat steps 3 and 4 until full comprehension/demonstration obtained

Adapted from Teachable Moments: Teach Back/

Two remedies for health literacy in the correctional setting, then, are to use simple everyday language when talking to the patient and to allow adequate time for the interaction (Nielsen-Bohlman et al., 2004). Experts advocate the following components in key verbal communications (Agency for Healthcare Research and Quality [AHRQ], 2010).

- Warm greeting
- Eye contact
- Slow down
- Limit content
- Teach-back

- Repeat key points
- Patient participation
- Plain, non-medical language
- Use graphics when explaining

Illness has meaning both biologically and in human experience. As cultural background has a huge impact on health literacy and interpretation of health care communication, care providers must pay attention to the predominant cultures of the patient population. Anthropologists list several cultural determinants of health care interpretation that can vary among groups (Nielsen-Bohlman et al., 2004).

- How a medical complaint is described

- How specifically a medical complaint is described

- Level of anxiety over the meaning of symptoms

- Relative focus on various body organs

- Engagement and response to therapies

Encouraging Medication Adherence

Patients also have a role in patient safety by adhering to the medical regimen – especially medication adherence - yet research indicates that half of the general patient population does not correctly self-administer medications (Brown & Bussell, 2011). Lack of medication adherence causes unnecessary patient deaths and at least 10% of hospitalizations in the US annually (DiMatteo, Giordani, Lepper, & Croghan, 2002). A focus on improving medication adherence among the incarcerated patient population can reduce mortality, morbidity, and clinical error.

Little is known about medication adherence among the incarcerated, although it would be expected to be similar or even lower than in the general population based on demographic indicators (Shelton, Ehret, Wakai, Kapetanovic, & Moran, 2010). As patient medication adherence is a key factor in treatment outcomes, it is an important consideration in efforts to improve patient safety.

Demographic indicators for low medical adherence include low health literacy (discussed above), poor patient motivation, and limited understanding of the disease process. Lack of social support and low socioeconomic status were also found to be indicators of reduced adherence (Brown & Bussell, 2011). Poor mental health is another indicator for non-adherence. Depression and anxiety, disorders disproportionately prevalent in the inmate population, reduce constancy in self-administering chronic care medications (Kronish et al., 2006).

Factors related to the particular disease process can decrease medication adherence (Kardas, Lewek, & Matyjaszczyk, 2013). Treating asymptomatic conditions such as hypertension can be difficult, especially if there are side effects to the medications. Even clinical improvement can reduce medication adherence. Patients are less motivated to continue medication when symptoms improve. The duration of illness affects medication adherence, with chronic conditions being the least motivating.

Although research is available on determinants of non-adherence, effective methods to improve patient medication adherence remain elusive (van Dulmen et al., 2007). Based on determinants of non-adherence (Brown & Bussell, 2011), a correctional setting can apply the following suggestions for improving adherence.

- Empower the patient by encouraging active involvement in treatment decisions such as, when possible, the time of day for medication administration. If the medication is a once-daily dose, the patient may prefer the evening pill line over the morning pill line based on sleep cycle. If the medication is self-administered through a keep-on-person program, discuss medication dosing options that fit the work and recreation schedule of the patient.

- Have all members of the health team reinforce names and effects of medications, and repeat health information and goals of treatment.

- Avoid changing numerous medications or treatment regimens in one time period. Gradually add or change medications, when possible, if the change requires behavior modification on the part of the patient.

- Encourage a "no shame" environment regarding literacy. Look for cues that the patient is unable to read, and alter information methods to accommodate findings such as using graphics and verbal explanations.

- Consider the ongoing economic impact of medication decisions. Patients will need to be able to continue to finance medication upon release.

Several additional interventions from other sources show support for effectiveness and promise for application in the correctional setting.

- Improved physician communication positively correlates with patient adherence (Haskard Zolnierek & DiMatteo, 2009). Efforts to enhance communication skills among correctional physicians could improve medication adherence. This can be supported organizationally by providing time for communication during the physician visit and improving provider skills in the use of teach-back methods when prescribing new medication regimens.

- Education, along with behavioral support, improved medication adherence in a systematic review of interventions with the chronically ill (Viswanathan et al., 2012). At least one prison has had positive outcomes for group education and peer support of patients with a chronic condition such as diabetes (Conrad & Delgado, 2010).

- Reminders for self-administration of medications were also effective in several studies among patients with chronic conditions, especially the aging (Viswanathan et al., 2012). Care providers should counsel patients to set up a reminder system for medication self-administration. Ideas include linking to an already-habituated daily activity like teeth-brushing or bedtime rituals, or creating a simple calendar to mark off for daily self-medication.

Applying Motivational Interviewing Principles

Motivational interviewing is a patient-centered style of communication designed to strengthen a patient's personal motivation for commitment to a specific goal through empathetic, non-confrontational dialog (Miller & Rollnick, 2013). It is popular in drug and alcohol treatment programs and often applied to health care goals such as smoke cessation and depression treatment adherence (Adelman & Myhre, 2013; Balán, Moyers, & Lewis-Fernández, 2013). Motivational interviewing involves five principles (Table 4. 5) to move an individual through the stages of change identified by the trans-theoretical model (Table 4.6).

Motivational interviewing may be helpful in engaging patients to adhere to therapy and be a part of the health care team. Systematic reviews of the use of this communication program in primary care populations (Vanbuskirk & Wetherell, 2013) and medical settings (Lundahl et al., 2013) indicate a modest advantage toward use of the technique. The extensive steps in the process, however, may limit usability in situations where there is limited time with the patient, such as a jail setting. Chronic care clinic visits in a long-term prison setting might benefit from motivational interviewing interventions across multiple appointments.

To assist with use of motivational interviewing principles in brief encounters, such as an emergency room, Yale University developed the Brief Negotiated Interview (BNI) that takes as little as seven minutes (Table 4.7). This tool has shown success when used with adolescent drinkers admitted to the emergency room following a car crash (D'Onofrio et al., 2012).

Using Patient Complaints/Inmate Grievances

Non-correctional health care systems have a formal mechanism for patients to report care concerns to the organization. Patient complaints across many aspects of care focus on the patient's identification of safety concerns. The inmate grievance process is the standard mechanism for incarcerated patients to report complaints and concerns about their health care system. Every correctional setting should include inmate grievances as part of the risk management process. Grievances can also serve as an early warning system for patient safety concerns. Correctional health care experts advocate for the inclusion of grievance review and response in an organization's patient safety program (Stern, Greifinger, & Mellow, 2010). Both individual and aggregate review of inmate health care grievances can reveal possible barriers to care provision and repetitive concerns that indicate a pattern in need of attention (Greifinger, 2012).

A comprehensive system incorporates patient complaints with other incident data for a more complete picture of patient safety status (Levtzion-Korach et al., 2010). This can be challenging as it requires attention to a category system that aligns

Table 4.5 Five Principles of Motivational Interviewing

Principle	Description
Express Empathy	• Empathy and acceptance encourages change
Develop Discrepancy	• Provide information showing a discrepancy between present behavior and important health goals
Avoid Argumentation	• Arguments are not productive and can lead to defensiveness and further resistance
Roll with Resistance	• Avoid directly opposing resistance • Present new perspectives but don't impose them
Support Self-Efficacy	• Encourage belief in the possibility of change • Keep responsibility for change with the patient • Encourage hope in use of range of actions

Adapted from Center for Substance Abuse Treatment, 2012

Table 4.6 Stages of Change Based on the Trans-Theoretical Model

Stage	Description
Pre-Contemplation	• No consideration of change
Contemplation	• Problem awareness • Slight consideration of stopping
Preparation	• Advantages of change and consequences of continuing undesirable behavior begin to outweigh advantages of continuing behavior
Action	• Begin to pursue strategies for change
Maintenance	• Behavior has been changed for more than six months. Strategies used to prevent reoccurrences.
Recurrence/ Permanent Exit	• Recurrence in early cycles is common and does not always indicate an abandonment of commitment • Success is indicated by permanent recovery

Adapted from Center for Substance Abuse Treatment, 2012

Table 4.7. Steps in the Brief Negotiated Interview

Step	Description
Raise the Subject	Establish rapport and raise the issue (medication compliance, smoking, treatment adherence)
Provide Feedback	Review the current status and compare with expected outcome such as end-organ damage, cancer, infection
Enhance Motivation	Assess readiness to change
Negotiate and Advise	Negotiate a goal with the patient and provide advice for ways to accomplish the goal

Adapted from D'Onofrio, Pantalon, Degutis, Fiellin, & O'Connor, 2005

patient complaints with staff incident reporting; however, a consistent use of standard terminology allows for better aggregate data analysis and, therefore, safety improvement (see also the inmate grievance management section in Chapter 1).

Correctional health care organizations that see the value of patient involvement in safety encourage the use of mechanisms like an inmate grievance process. Experience in other settings indicates the following factors that encourage patient participation (Birks, Hall, Peat, & Watt, 2011).

- Including the patient's input when designing the system.

- Educating the patient about the system.

- Clearly identifying how the information was used to improve the system.

Obtaining patient input, providing patient awareness, and sharing outcomes of patient involvement through the inmate grievance system can improve health care delivery and reduce clinical error.

Summary

The role of patients in the correctional health care patient safety program may, at first, seem minimal. Applying principles of patient-centered care and educating the patient population about their role can, however, increase meaningful participation. Patients can be valuable members of their health care team when they understand their role, are health-literate and are motivated. Health professionals have an obligation to encourage patient participation to improve safety and reduce clinical error.

References

Adelman, W. & Myhre, K.E. (2013). *Motivational Interviewing: Helping Teenaged Smokers to Quit.* Retrieved from http://contemporarypediatrics.modern medicine.com/contemporary-pediatrics/news/motivational-interviewing-helping-teenaged-smokers-quit?page=0,4

Agency for Healthcare Research and Quality (AHRQ). (2010). *Health literacy universal precautions toolkit. AHRQ Publication No. 10-0046-EF.* Agency for Healthcare Research and Quality. U.S. Department of Health and Human Services. Retrieved from www.nchealthliteracy.org/toolkit/

Amodeo, A., Jin, Y., & Kling, J. (2009). Preparing for life beyond prison walls: The literacy of incarcerated adults near release. *Computer, 16*(14), 70.

Balán, I.C., Moyers, T.B., & Lewis-Fernández, R. (2013). Motivational pharmacotherapy: Combining motivational interviewing and antidepressant therapy to improve treatment adherence. *Psychiatry: Interpersonal & Biological Processes, 76*(3), 203–209.

Birks, Y., Hall, J., Peat, M., & Watt, I. (2011). Promoting patient involvement in safety initiatives. *Nursing Management, 18*(1), 16–20.

Brown, M.T. & Bussell, J.K. (2011). Medication adherence: WHO cares? *Mayo Clinic Proceedings, 86*(4), 304–314. doi:10.4065/mcp.2010.0575

Center for Substance Abuse Treatment. (2012). *Enhancing motivation for change in substance abuse treatment.* Substance Abuse and Mental Health Services Administration. Retrieved from www.ncbi.nlm.nih.gov/books/NBK64967/pdf/TOC.pdf

Conrad, M. & Delgado, M. (2010, September). *Taking control of your health in the New Jersey prison system.* National Council on Aging Webinar. Retrieved from www.ncoa.org/improve-health/center-for-healthy-aging/content-library/Sept-2010-Special-Webinar-Prison-Powerpoint.pdf

Cornett, S. (2009). Assessing and addressing health literacy. *Online Journal of Issues in Nursing, 14* (3), manuscript 2. Retrieved from www.nursingworld.org/MainMenuCategories/ANAMarketplace/ANAPeriodic als/OJIN/TableofContents/Vol142009/No3Sept09/Assessing-Health-Literacy-.aspx

D'Onofrio, G., Fiellin, D.A., Pantalon, M.V., Chawarski, M.C., Owens, P.H., Degutis, L.C., … O'Connor, P.G. (2012). A brief intervention reduces hazardous and harmful drinking in emergency department patients. *Annals of Emergency Medicine, 60*(2), 181–192. doi:10.1016/j.annemergmed.2012.02.006

D'Onofrio, G., Pantalon, M.V., Degutis, L.C., Fiellin, D.A., & O'Connor, P.G. (2005). *The Yale Brief Negotiated Interveiw Manual.* New Haven, CT: Yale University School of Medicine.

DiMatteo, M.R., Giordani, P.J., Lepper, H.S., & Croghan, T.W. (2002). Patient adherence and medical treatment outcomes: A meta-analysis. *Medical Care, 40*(9), 794–811. doi:10.1097/01.MLR.0000024612. 61915.2D

Emanuel, L., Berwick, D., Conway, J., Combes, J., Hatlie, M., Leape, L., ... Walton, M. (2008). What exactly is patient safety. *Advances in Patient Safety: New Directions and Alternative Approaches, 1*. Retrieved from http://ahrq.hhs. gov/downloads/pub/advances2/vol1/Advances-Emanuel-Berwick_110.pdf

Entwistle, V.A., Mello, M.M., & Brennan, T.A. (2005). Advising patients about patient safety: Current initiatives risk shifting responsibility. *Joint Commission Journal on Quality and Patient Safety / Joint Commission Resources, 31*(9), 483–494.

Epstein, R.M., Fiscella, K., Lesser, C.S., & Stange, K.C. (2010). Why the nation needs a policy push on patient-centered health care. *Health Affairs, 29*(8), 1489–1495. doi:10.1377/hlthaff.2009.0888

Greenberg, E., Dunleavy, E., & Kutner, M. (2007). *Literacy Behind Bars: Results from the 2003 National Assessment of Adult Literacy Prison Survey.* U.S. Department of Education. Retrieved from http://nces.ed.gov/pubs2007/2007473.pdf

Greifinger, R.B. (2012). Independent review of clinical health services for prisoners. *International Journal of Prisoner Health, 8*(3), 141–150. doi:10.1108/17449201211285012

Hickson, G.B., Clayton, E.W., Githens, P.B., & Sloan, F.A. (1992). Factors that prompted families to file medical malpractice claims following perinatal injuries. *JAMA: The Journal of the American Medical Association, 267*(10), 1359–1363.

Holme, A. (2009). Exploring the role of patients in promoting safety: Policy to practice. *British Journal of Nursing, 18*(22), 1392–1395.

Institute for Patient- and Family-Centered Care (IPFCC). (n.d.). *Patient- and family-centered care.* Retrieved from www.ipfcc.org/pdf/CoreConcepts.pdf

Institute of Medicine (2001). *Crossing the quality chasm: A new health system for the 21st century.* Washington, D.C.: National Academy Press. Retrieved from http://search.ebscohost.com/login.aspx?direct=true&scope=site&db=nlebk&db=nlabk&AN=86916

Kardas, P., Lewek, P., & Matyjaszczyk, M. (2013). Determinants of patient adherence: A review of systematic reviews. *Frontiers in Pharmacology, 4*. doi:10.3389/fphar.2013.00091

Kripalani, S., Bengtzen, R., Henderson, L.E., & Jacobson, T.A. (2008). Clinical research in low-literacy populations: Using teach-back to assess comprehension of informed consent and privacy information. *IRB: Ethics and Human Research, 30*(2), 13–19.

Kronish, I.M., Rieckmann, N., Halm, E.A., Shimbo, D., Vorchheimer, D., Haas, D.C., & Davidson, K.W. (2006). Persistent depression affects adherence to secondary prevention behaviors after acute coronary syndromes. *Journal of General Internal Medicine, 21*(11), 1178–1183. doi:10.1111/j.1525-1497.2006.00586.x

Levtzion-Korach, O., Frankel, A., Alcalai, H., Keohane, C., Orav, J., Graydon-Baker, E., ... Tomov, E.I. (2010). Integrating incident data from five reporting systems to assess patient safety: Making sense of the elephant. *Joint Commission Journal on Quality and Patient Safety, 36*(9), 402–410.

Lundahl, B., Moleni, T., Burke, B.L., Butters, R., Tollefson, D., Butler, C., & Rollnick, S. (2013). Motivational interviewing in medical care settings: A systematic review and meta-analysis of randomized controlled trials. *Patient Education and Counseling, 93*(2), 157–168. doi:10.1016/j.pec.2013.07.012

McLaughlin, G.H. (1969). SMOG grading: A new readability formula. *Journal of Reading, 12*(8), 639–646.

Miller, Chung, M., Connell, A.M., Lennie, T.A., & Moser, D.K. (2012). Abstract 16038: Health literacy predicts cardiovascular risk in the male prison population. *Circulation, 126*, A16038.

Miller, W.R., & Rollnick, S. (2013). *Motivational interviewing: Helping people change* (3rd ed.). New York, NY: Guilford Press.

Nielsen-Bohlman, L., Panzer, A.M., & Kindig, D.A. (2004). *Health literacy: A prescription to end confusion*. Washington, D.C.: National Academies Press. Retrieved from http://site.ebrary.com/id/10062734

Paris, J. (2006). Interaction between correctional staff and health care providers in the delivery of medical care. In M. Puisis (Ed.), *Clinical practice in correctional medicine* (pp. 12-18). Philadelphia, PA: Mosby Elsevier.

Pearlmutter, M. (2011). Physician apologies and general admissions of gault: Amending the federal rules of evidence. *Ohio State Law Journal, 72*(3), 687-722.

Peat, M., Entwistle, V., Hall, J., Birks, Y., Golder, S., & on behalf of the PIPS Group. (2010). Scoping review and approach to appraisal of interventions intended to involve patients in patient safety. *Journal of Health Services Research & Policy, 15*(suppl 1), 17–25. doi:10.1258/jhsrp.2009.009040

Pelling, M.H. (2004). Engaging patients in safety: Barriers and solutions. In P.L. Spath (Ed.), *Partnering with Patients to Reduce Medical errors* (pp. 85-108). Chicago, IL: Health Forum.

Robbennolt, J. K. (2009). Apologies and medical error. *Clinical Orthopedic Related Research, 467*, 376-382.

Saxton, J.W. & Finkelstein, M.M. (2004). Enabling patient involvement without increasing liability risk. In P.L. Spath (Ed.), *Partnering with patients to reduce medical errors* (pp.109-140). Chicago, IL: Health Forum.

Shelton, D., Ehret, M.J., Wakai, S., Kapetanovic, T., & Moran, M. (2010). Psychotropic medication adherence in correctional facilities: A review of the literature. *Journal of Psychiatric and Mental Health Nursing, 17*(7), 603–613. doi:10.1111/j.1365-2850.2010.01587.x

Spath, P. (2004). Safety from the patient's point of view. In P.L. Spath (Ed.), *Partnering with patients to reduce medical errors* (pp. 1-34). Chicago, IL: Health Forum.

Stern, M.F., Greifinger, R.B., & Mellow, J. (2010). Patient safety: Moving the bar in prison health care standards. *American Journal of Public Health, 100*(11), 2103.

Teachable moments: Teach back/show back method. (2011). *Patient Education Management, 18*(12), 145.

The Joint Commission (TJC). (2013). Facts about Speak-Up. Retrieved from www.jointcommission.org/assets/1/6/Facts_Speak_Up.pdf

US Department of Health & Human Services (HHS). (2009). *Simply put: A guide for creating easy-to-understand materials* (3rd ed.). Atlanta, GA: Centers for Disease Control and Prevention.

Van Dulmen, S., Sluijs, E., van Dijk, L., de Ridder, D., Heerdink, R., & Bensing, J. (2007). Patient adherence to medical treatment: A review of reviews. *BMC Health Services Research, 7*(1), 55. doi:10.1186/1472-6963-7-55

Vanbuskirk, K.A. & Wetherell, J.L. (2013). Motivational interviewing with primary care populations: A systematic review and meta-analysis. *Journal of Behavioral Medicine.* doi:10.1007/s10865-013-9527-4

Vincent, C.A. & Coulter, A. (2002). Patient safety: What about the patient? *Quality and Safety in Health Care, 11*(1), 76–80.

Viswanathan, M., Golin, C.E., Jones, C.D., Ashok, M., Blalock, S.J., Wines, R.C., … Lohr, K.N. (2012). Interventions to improve adherence to self-administered medications for chronic diseases in the United States: A systematic review. *Annals of Internal Medicine, 157*(11), 785–795.

Wachter, R.M. (2012). *Understanding patient safety.* New York, NY: McGraw Hill Medical.

Weiner, S.J., Schwartz, A., Sharma, G., Binns-Calvey, A., Ashley, N., Kelly, B., … Harris, I. (2013). Patient-centered decision making and health care outcomes: An observational study. *Annals of Internal Medicine, 158*(8), 573–579. doi:10.7326/0003-4819-158-8-201304160-00001

Weiss, D. (2007). *Health Literacy and Patient Safety: Help Patients Understand* (2nd ed.). Chicago, IL: American Medical Association. Retrieved from www.ama-assn.org/ama1/pub/upload/mm/367/healthlitclinicians.pdf

White, M., Garbez, R., Carroll, M., Brinker, E., & Howie-Esquivel, J. (2013). Is "teach-back" associated with knowledge retention and hospital readmission in hospitalized heart failure patients? *The Journal of Cardiovascular Nursing, 28*(2), 137–146. doi:10.1097/JCN.0b013e31824987bd

Zolnierek, K.B.H. & DiMatteo, M.R. (2009). Physician communication and patient adherence to treatment: A meta-analysis. *Medical Care, 47*(8), 826–834. doi:10.1097/MLR.0b013e31819a5acc

5 Health Care Workers

The first concern when investigating a clinical error is often the performance of the individual staff worker closest to the error. As displayed in the Patient Safety Model (Figure 5.1), the worker functions alongside systems to deliver efficient and effective patient care. True, staff involved in a clinical error may have accountability and a Just Culture within an organization supports the need for evaluating staff accountability along with other factors in unraveling error cause; often, though, staff are a second victim in an error outcome. The concepts of Just Culture and second victim are discussed in Chapter 2.

Competency is the most important principle to consider within the domain of health care workers (Table 5.1). Staff skilled in specific functions reduce the risk of clinical errors and thus improve patient safety. Internal and external sources of stress may compromise workers' abilities to think clearly or act responsibly. Correctional health care experts have described the need to train staff on patient safety, evaluate competency in professional practice annually, and address staff-centric issues such as fatigue and burnout (Stern, Greifinger, & Mellow, 2010).

Figure 5.1 A Patient Safety Model of Health Care

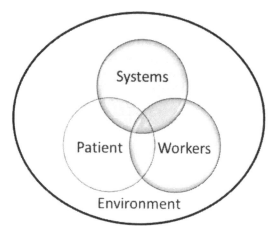

Adapted from Emanuel et al., 2008

Competent Care Providers

Competent care demands competent providers; however, their recruitment is a challenge. Despite the modern, improved perceptions in some quarters, clinicians are still reluctant to seek work in correctional settings. Efforts to engage a competent health care workforce must start with a positive and enthusiastic attitude at the employee search and interview stage.

All new staff members need a thorough and professional orientation to the unique aspects of health care delivery in a secure setting. Leadership and management should not assume that new hires with past corrections experience are necessarily properly trained for their current jobs. It is crucial that managers do not feel pressured by staff shortages or rapid turnover to unduly shorten the training period. There can be no allowance for failing to validate new employees' competencies before having them work independently.

Table 5.1 Domains and Principles of Patient Safety

Domain of Patient Safety	Principle of Patient Safety
Environment of Care	A Just Culture in a Learning Organization
Systems for Therapeutic Action	High Reliability System Design Communication and Teamwork
Recipient of Care	Patient-Centered Care
Health Care Workers	Competent Care Providers

Following this initial validation, staff should receive continuing competency training in a clinical setting of rapid change. Ongoing training and peer review in small facilities can be difficult. In a review of root causes of sentinel events reported to The Joint Commission (TJC) from 1995 to 2004, lack of staff orientation and training was a top cause of clinical error, second only to communication, in traditional settings (TJC, 2005). Health care leaders need to regularly remind all team members that they are accountable for safe practice and for continuing professional development. Organizations should also be held accountable for monitoring fatigue, burnout, and workforce issues to ensure adequate staffing (staff-to-patient ratios) and good employee morale, as all of these conditions are found to affect patient safety.

Pre-Employment Evaluation

Each position in an organization requires baseline skills and credentials. Job descriptions should specify the minimum requirements to perform in the role, along with desirable qualities that would make a candidate stand out. A well-crafted job description is helpful in creating a short list of possible candidates from among applicants. It is tempting to set the bar at a low level, especially in an organization with high turnover and low desirability. But this is a short-sighted action. Hiring poorly-qualified staff increases safety risk in an already risky environment.

"Applicants often appear superbly qualified during their interview yet cannot function adequately on the job. Thus, I consider the probation period an extension of the interview process offered to a select few who are worth the investment of salary while being observed for competence at work. I am able to determine that a new hire is made of the right stuff by closely observing his or her performance during the first two weeks of patient care.

I recall a physician who seemed well-trained and highly motivated at the start; but within the first two weeks problems with his work appeared. He arrived in clinic late and then worked too slowly to see the line of patients before the prison yard needed to be shut down for the evening. He was either abrupt or non-communicative in dealing with patients and staff. He was sloppy. He generally appeared disheveled in a dirty white coat. His diagnoses were incomplete and inaccurate; his planned treatments contrary to best practices.

One would think dismissal of this employee was a "no brainer." But there is no such thing as an easy dismissal. If the employee understood his or her failings then we would never see the lapses. So it is likely that as a poor fit as this physician was for the job, he would deny being unable or incompetent to do it. Therefore observing his inadequate performance was barely half my job. It remained for me to document my findings in writing, present this writing to the employee with a witness, give him time to improve, write up the results of his work following the first assessment, present those findings to him, and then inform him of a decision to terminate employment if he was unable to meet the reasonable expectations provided to him.

Even after all of that I was prepared for a lawsuit for wrongful termination; but keeping a person on the job so ill-suited for the work will lead to patient harm and lawsuits as well. It was better for all that this physician be told to find work elsewhere. He complained. His wife called me to complain. But I held my ground. It was the right thing to do." - **Bruce P. Barnett, MD, JD, MBA**

Once hiring supervisors determine that an individual has the qualifications to meet the job description, credentialing will validate that the candidate has met all licensure and certification requirements. Online databases for validating unencumbered licensure have eased the process, but it can still be time-consuming to determine that potential hires actually have the licensure and certification qualifications that they claim. Some settings validate credentials only after an

interview process determines that the individual is desirable for the position. Some even wait until after the person has accepted the position. Unfortunately, at this point, there are also some who take the word of the individual and do not validate licensure and certification. This can lead to unsafe patient care. In some quarters, the correctional setting is still considered an easy location for poor or unethical practitioners to find employment. The National Practitioner Data Bank can provide information on closed and settled claims history. The smartest and safest option is to verify credentials for every new hire before the first day of employment and then to require a continued valid and unencumbered licensure for the entire duration of employment.

The interview process is a good place to start in establishing a patient safety perspective for new employees. Once the candidate's background has been vetted, a face-to-face interview is usually arranged, although some systems perform a phone interview first. The interview process is not only an opportunity to evaluate the candidate; it also establishes organizational priorities for the potential new employee. The interviewer's description of the process of health care delivery in the organization establishes the foundation for the professional's practice in the setting. Therefore, the interviewer should include principles of patient safety and error reduction as a part of the interview dialog.

Behavioral interviewing is a popular means of interviewing candidates for clinical positions that require critical thinking and clinical judgment skills. This interviewing process engages the candidate in describing past behaviors and experiences that indicate they have the knowledge, skills and attitudes necessary to be successful in the open position (Broscio, 2013). Behavioral interviewing is based on the concept that the best predictor of future performance is past performance. This can be accomplished by including least one patient safety scenario in the behavioral interviewing question list. Here are some examples that can be modified for use in a variety of correctional settings.

- Have you ever had a conflict with a co-worker? How did you resolve it?

- Have you ever made a clinical error? What did you do about it?

- Explain what you have done when you disagreed with a team member about a course of action or treatment with a patient you were involved with.

Most hiring processes also include a reference check. This can be an opportunity to ask prior work colleagues about the patient safety practices of potential new employees. Here again, teamwork and conflict resolution skills play a major role in patient safety and can be asked of an employment reference. Honesty, accountability and patient-centered behaviors are all indicators of safe patient practices.

Initial Orientation and Ongoing Competency

A patient safety emphasis continues once a clinician is hired. The orientation period is an opportunity to build on the foundation of safe practice but can, unfortunately, also abound with bad habits and shoddy practices. Short-staffed and harried health care programs may rely solely on having new employees read policies and shadow available staff as a method for initial orientation to a position. A structured orientation program that emphasizes core competencies and prioritizes safe delivery of patient care is essential to reduce clinical risk.

From the start of employment, staff members need to know and consistently use the processes and systems that support safe practice, as well as know how to engage the organization when there is a breach in the system. Orientation to the organization should indicate the importance of patient safety as a part of everyone's job description. Correctional health care experts suggest that key principles of error reduction be a part of initial and ongoing staff training (Stern et al., 2010).

Shelton, Weiskopf, and Nicholson (2010) provide a five-phase competency program model for correctional nursing staff that includes four to six weeks of close supervision followed by a year of mentoring. Although some may consider this timeframe extensive, the need for competency in a variety of clinical areas – along with acclimation to the unique criminal justice environment – requires extensive knowledge, skills and attitudes. Depending on the setting, correctional health care workers deliver care requiring competency in acute care, community health, emergency, geriatric, maternity, psychiatric and hospice practice (Shelton, Weiskopf, & Nicholson, 2010). A competency program of structured supervised experiences followed by lengthy mentorship could be created for other correctional health disciplines, as well.

Simulation exercises are an effective way to develop and maintain competent clinical practice. Simulation exercises allow for deliberate practice and then reflection on risky patient procedures. These exercises can be created to focus on vulnerable processes such as emergency response, team communication, and system changes (Schmidt, Goldhaber-Fiebert, Ho, & McDonald, 2013). They also help staff practice new procedures in a safe environment without fear of patient harm during skill development. This is a great improvement over the classic model of "see one, do one, teach one." Research in professional education indicates that using simulations improves knowledge and clinical reasoning (Cook, Erwin, & Triola, 2010; McGaghie, Issenberg, Cohen, Barsuk, & Wayne, 2011).

A form of simulation in correctional settings is the use of man-down and disaster drills. These experiences allow staff members to practice skills needed for high-risk, and often infrequent, situations that require both clinical and communication skills. Following the simulation, holding debriefing sessions maximizes the value of these learning experiences by allowing for reflection and course correction, both organizationally and individually. Unfortunately, these drills rarely focus on team communication and interactive skills so necessary for patient safety. Blum and colleagues (2005) successfully used the simulation experience to practice such communication skills as speaking up when direction is questioned and the use of the two-challenge rule (both discussed in Chapter 3). Correctional settings would benefit from adding a team communication objective to man-down and disaster simulations, along with a more robust debriefing component. Clinical practice simulations are just beginning in correctional health care. A system of nursing competency simulations is in development in the Connecticut state prison system with potential for use in other systems (Diaz, Panosky & Shelton, 2014).

Accountability

Health care professionals have both ethical and legal accountability for their practices. Individual accountability for professional practice is a basic principle of a just patient safety culture (discussed in Chapter 2). Ethical accountability is defined in professional practice codes, such as the American Nurses Association (ANA) Code for Nurses and the World Medical Association (WMA) Code of Medical Ethics, as a commitment to the public to provide health care in the best interests of the patient (ANA, 2001; WMA, 2006). Practical application of this duty to patients includes care and concern for patient safety in the decisions and actions taken on their behalf. This is embedded within the central tenet of medical practice to "above all do no harm." The movement toward professional accountability to learn from error, however, and an explicit accountability for safety practices, is just beginning (Emanuel et al., 2008).

Correctional health care professionals are also guided by specialty ethical codes such as the Society of Correctional Physicians Code of Ethics (SCP, n.d.) and the American Correctional Health Services Association Ethics Statement (ACHSA, n.d.). Both documents confirm the need for correctional practitioners to be accountable to respect human dignity and prevent harm when engaged in patient care.

Scope of practice. Boundaries of various licensed health care providers can be different among state practice acts. Practicing within the scope of practice of each profession is a safety measure. Licensing boards establish boundaries of practice and determine the elements of treatment that providers can perform on or for the patient. Scope of practice is based on the verifiable knowledge and skills of the professional, as determined by licensing standards. A primary role of licensing and practice acts is to guard the public safety (Russell, 2012).

In the correctional setting, scope-of-practice boundaries can become blurred as well-meaning staff attempt to accomplish needed care in a low-resource environment. Clinical error can result when staff members must make decisions or perform functions beyond their education, experience and – more importantly – licensure. A major patient safety measure, then, is to confirm that all post duties are within the scope of practice of the individual assigned to the position. Also important is ongoing education regarding expectations for staff to practice within their licensure and question assignments that go beyond that boundary.

A review of closed legal claims specific to nursing practice found that scope-of-practice issues were a small percentage of claim volume but held the highest average indemnity payment (Benton & Flynn, 2013). This could be due to jury perception that practicing outside of legal boundary is a particularly significant breach of licensure. Recommendations to protect against scope-of-practice claims are to: 1) create policy, procedure and protocol based on state scope-of-practice parameters; 2) enhance professional written and spoken communication skills; 3) maintain clinical competencies related to the needs of the patient population and specialty; and 4) establish an effective chain of command that is initiated when the necessary care exceeds licensure boundaries of local staff (Benton & Flynn, 2013).

Behavioral concepts of human error. Four behavioral concepts of human error have been identified as a means to evaluate individual accountability when patient safety is jeopardized or clinical error takes place (Marx, 2001). They help in determining if the health care provider's risk-taking actions were intentional or inadvertent. These concepts include negligent conduct, reckless conduct, and knowing violations each of which require some action to prevent future risk. The need to address behaviors that contribute to safety issues is a fundamental part of a Just Culture addressed in Chapter 2.

Working along a continuum of intentionality, an adverse event resulting from "human error" does not ascribe intent or even a departure from the usual standards or care. The label of "negligent conduct" indicates the error at issue was unreasonable or preventable as the practitioner should have known the risk of the mistaken action. Even further into intentionality is "reckless conduct", in which the individual did know the risk of the mistaken behavior and thus had a conscious disregard for the consequences. If an evaluation determines that negligent or reckless conduct caused the error, sanction can protect patients from further harm. In an employment setting, this can involve progressive discipline or termination. From a legal perspective, this may involve license suspension or revocation. It can be a tricky balance to encourage open reporting of error or risky clinical situations while also taking action to remove truly negligent practitioners from patient care situations.

In the case of human error, where intentionality is not a factor, differentiating errors as skill-based, rule-based or knowledge-based can determine practitioner-based causality (Spath, 2011).

Skill-based errors. Skill-based errors involve a slip or lapse in automatic activities that are not ordinarily preventable but will occur from time to time because humans (and even machines) are not perfect. Causes of errors that occur despite best application of skills include distractions, fatigue, or stress. An experienced provider automates many actions of practice and performs them habitually and subconsciously, much like safety activities in driving a car. Skill-based errors can happen when habituated activities in normal conditions are not able to overcome condition changes. In the car example, driving speeds adequate for taking bends during normal road conditions are inadequate for maintaining safety in a heavy rainstorm. By way of comparison, driving too fast on a patch of unexpected "black ice" is human error, whereas failure to reduce speed in the rain is negligence. In a medical situation, a provider error is not negligence if the particular condition would not likely be recognized by most colleagues awakened by a call from the nurse. System mechanisms, such as process checklists, can help reduce skill-based human errors (Bohne & Peruzzi, 2010).

Rule-based errors. On the other hand, rule-based errors are usually preventable mistakes. Health care practitioners manage many clinical decisions by activating rules of practice (Spath, 2011). Yet, the wrong rule can be applied to determine a course of action. This might happen due to the ambiguous nature of the situation or an inadequate presentation of information. A rule-based error could also include the intentional over-riding of a known rule due to the emergent nature of a situation. For example, a nurse may give one patient another patient's medication during a hypertensive crisis when there is no stock medication available.

Knowledge-based errors. Knowledge-based errors happen when practitioners are not prepared to face a new situation (Spath, 2011). Health care staff entering the correctional environment may have limited experience with the vast number of conditions or treatments provided in a secure setting. These errors are also usually preventable. Orientation and ongoing competency validation go a long way toward reducing knowledge-based errors, but staff also need to know how to access advanced knowledge when they are unsure of an action. This can include awareness of how to access clinical references, policies, procedure manuals, and management staff on all shifts and days of the week.

Issues Internal to Health Care Workers

Individual characteristics and life situations of health care staff can affect patient safety. Although employees certainly have a right to choose their lifestyle outside of patient care hours, lifestyle decisions and situations can adversely affect the ability to deliver safe patient care. Several practitioner characteristics can increase the likelihood of clinical error and may require organizational intervention.

General Mental and Physical Health

The health of individual workers affects patient safety, as an unwell employee is less able to maintain the level of vigilance, critical thinking, and physical stamina needed to provide quality care (Trinkoff et al., 2008). Feeling unwell, depressed, or anxious negatively affects mental processes and therefore can contribute to clinical error. Battling even mild illness, such as cold or flu, can lead to sleep difficulty and ensuing fatigue. Over-the-counter cold preparations can fog thinking and slow mental processing. Health care staff must be able to clearly think and respond to changing situations during care delivery. This ability to quickly respond and change course can be blunted by both the health condition and the treatments being used for it.

The general aging process or chronic disease can make it difficult for professionals to maintain the cognitive or motor skills necessary to safely perform their patient care responsibilities. Every health care organization should have policy and procedure for determining when a staff member is sufficiently impaired from being able to perform job duties and the actions that need to be taken to relieve them of their duties. At the same time, of course, organizations must meet appropriate licensing board issues and comply with the Americans with Disabilities Act (Hoffman, 2009).

Fatigue

The long-studied relationship of staff fatigue and clinical error began with concern for the effect of disrupted circadian rhythms and interrupted sleep of interns and medical residents (Gaba & Howard, 2002). Fatigue can cause lapses in attention, difficulty staying focused, and reduced reaction time, making it difficult to respond to urgent and emergent patient needs. It also can affect communication, motivation, and irritability, thus reducing smooth team interactions. Impeded problem-solving and information-processing also disrupts cognitive functioning and diagnostic abilities. This increases the risk of clinical error and adverse patient events (TJC, 2012). Correctional health care experts identify preventing staff fatigue and burnout as a key patient safety measure (Stern et al., 2010).

The individual staff member, as well as the health care organization, has responsibilities regarding monitoring and reducing worker fatigue in order to increase patient safety. Staff members must obtain adequate rest prior to a work shift. This may require adjustments in personal schedules to accommodate the need. Staff must also be willing to limit work hours to those that allow for adequate rest. This may involve reducing voluntary overtime. For example, the ANA considers it an ethical responsibility for nurses to consider their level of fatigue before accepting any assignment beyond the regularly scheduled workday or week (ANA, 2006).

The following measures can help staff members who are sleepy in the midst of a work shift.

- **Napping.** A 15-minute nap can increase alertness both during long shifts and over the night shift (Amin et al., 2012; Lovato & Lack, 2010; Milner & Cote, 2009). Many facilities prohibit napping but should reconsider this policy in the light of research findings. Instead, naps could be encouraged during breaks or meal periods when the staff member is totally free of clinical responsibilities (Rogers & Hughes, 2008).

- **Caffeine.** 200 mg (about 16 ounces of brewed coffee) increases performance and alertness within 15-30 minutes (Rogers & Hughes, 2008). Caffeine in combination with napping had an even greater effect on alertness (Schweitzer, Randazzo, Stone, Erman, & Walsh, 2006). Some organizations provide coffee as a part of services to staff members. Moderate caffeine intake can improve alertness, especially during shift work.

- Other interventions include bright lighting and exercise have been proposed, but studies have yielded mixed results (Rogers & Hughes, 2008).

Work Stress and Burnout

Work stress, in addition to fatigue, may lead to clinical error. Chronic work stress, coined "burnout" in the mid-1970s, comes from the emotional exhaustion of managing the ongoing stress of a high-pressured, constantly changing, conflict-rich workplace (Jennings, 2008). All employees do not respond to work stress in the same way. Challenges of balancing home and family lives also contribute to greater work stress (Bryant, Fairbrother, & Fenton, 2000; Gottlieb, Kelloway, & Martin-Matthews, 1996). A review of research on reduction of work stress in health care organizations supports the use of empowerment and social support to reduce stress. Although a relationship between moderation of work stress and increased patient safety may seem intuitive, evidence is not found for the link (Jennings, 2008). Nevertheless, correctional health care experts recommend a focus on reducing workplace stress and burnout to improve patient safety (Stern et al., 2010).

Compassion Fatigue and Vicarious Traumatization

While work stress and burnout can result from many workplace factors including organizational culture or lack of resources, compassion fatigue and vicarious traumatization are directly linked to the patient relationship. Health care workers regularly treat individuals in pain, suffering from debilitating disease and struggling with mental illness or under major life stress. This can be a major work stress that affects clinical decision-making and patient safety (Dunkley & Whelan, 2006).

Compassion fatigue, also called secondary traumatic stress, is described as a building distress over knowing about, and wanting to help, a traumatized or suffering person (Sabo, 2011). This can be a natural consequence of empathetic engagement in a therapeutic relationship. Those health care practitioners with high empathetic response to their patients are more likely to experience this condition (Adams, Boscarino, & Figley, 2006). The physical and psychological outcomes of compassion fatigue affect functioning, while the detachment and avoidance that ensues in an effort to avoid further stress can lead to poor performance.

Vicarious traumatization, like compassion fatigue, is an occupational stress for those who work with high-demand populations. Compassion fatigue may be a precursor to vicarious traumatization in the continuum of emotional stress. Both mirror post-traumatic stress disorder in symptoms (Sabo, 2011). Vicarious traumatization, however, expresses the distress that professionals experience through working specifically with patients who have been traumatized, and results from integrating the patient's experiences both psychologically and emotionally (Dunkley & Whelan, 2006).

Both compassion fatigue and vicarious traumatization have been extensively studied in the oncology, emergency, and hospice workplace settings (Sabo, 2011). Early work with correctional staff, specifically nurses, indicates a similar stress response when working with a patient population that is regularly traumatized by a highly controlled and depersonalized correctional system, while also having a high degree of past abuse and trauma. A survey of over 200 correctional nurses found that nearly two thirds of respondents scored at moderate or high risk of vicarious traumatization; this was more likely for nurses working in high security settings (Munger, 2013).

Reducing the impact of working with a traumatized patient population can lead to improved patient safety and staff health. Both individual and organizational interventions can succeed. Individual staff need an awareness of the threat of compassion fatigue and vicarious traumatization (Pross, 2006). This understanding can lead to a therapeutic self-awareness that may halt progression of the fatigue or traumatization before it takes hold through somatic and psychological manifestations. Boundaries in the provider-patient relationship are of particular importance in a correctional setting, where patients may have tendencies toward exploiting or deceiving those in a helper role. Maintaining a balance in working with both highly traumatized patients and more normalized patients can also be helpful (Pross, 2006). In a correctional setting, this may mean rotating through the various positions so that individual staff are not always working with the administrative segregation population, for example. From an organizational perspective, a supportive work environment decreases the perception of burnout and vicarious traumatization (Argentero & Setti, 2011). Organizational awareness and intervention can reduce staff emotional distress and subsequently reduce potential clinical error.

Drug or Alcohol Impairment

The number of physicians and nurses who have a substance abuse disorder is similar to the general public, although one might think that it should be less (K. B. Gold & Teitelbaum, 2010; Kunyk, 2013). The impact of working while impaired by drugs or alcohol as a health care professional, however, can be devastating. Excessive use of drugs or alcohol impairs an individual's cognitive processing and motor skills, making them more likely to perform a clinical error. Both the ANA (1984) and the American Medical Association (AMA; 2011) address the issue of impaired professionals, as does the American College of Healthcare Executives (ACHE; 2013). These professional associations understand the need to monitor and manage substance-impaired professionals to maintain a primary responsibility for safe patient care (Hoffman, 2009).

Health care staff need to know what impairment looks like so that action can be taken if a team member shows signs of needing assistance (Table 5.2). Health care workers have an ethical, and often legal, responsibility to report suspected drug or alcohol impairment in team members (Baldisseri, 2007). A policy and procedure should be in place to handle possibly impaired staff members, including reporting and treatment (Hoffman, 2009).

Table 5.2. Signs and Symptoms of Substance Involvement

Staff Actions	Physical Signs	Behavior Changes
• Brief, unexplained absences from the nursing unit • Rounding at odd hours • Medication errors • Isolation from peers • Mood changes after meals or breaks • Frequent reports of lack of pain relief from assigned patients • Narcotics obsession, offering to medicate a co-worker's patients • Wasted narcotics attributed to a single nurse • Increased narcotic sign-outs • Discrepancies with the narcotic record and/or the patient record • Decreased quality of care, arriving late to work, and requesting to leave early	• Shakiness and/or tremors • Fatigue • Slurred speech • Frequent use of mouthwash or breath mints • Watery eyes • Constricted/dilated pupils • Diaphoresis • Unsteady gait • Frequent runny nose • Weight gain or loss • Change in grooming	• Frequent mood changes • Outbursts of anger • Inappropriate laughter • Hyperactivity or hypoactivity • Lack of concentration • Blackout periods • Cold weather clothing in warm weather to hide track marks • Frequent accidents or emergencies • Personal relationship issues • Denial of the problem/ frequent lying • Decreased judgment in their own performance

Taken from Thomas & Siela, 2011, with permission

Issues External to Health Care Workers

Worker issues external to themselves include staffing patterns, turnover, and vacancies. These organizational situations can be particularly acute in a correctional setting where recruitment of highly-trained professionals is difficult. Shortages of various professional classes can put pressure on health care team members to "cover" for a vacancy, thus risking patient safety in order to get the job done. As discussed earlier, worker fatigue, which can be affected by staffing patterns or understaffing, contributes to increased clinical error. Correctional health experts also see a link between high staff vacancies, inadequate nursing staffing, and decreased patient safety (Stern et al., 2010).

Three components of staffing patterns should be considered when evaluating the staffing effect on patient safety: staffing ratios, staffing mix, and shift work rotation (Lundstrom, Pugliese, Bartley, Cox, & Guither, 2002).

- **Staffing ratios** – the number of staff per patient – has been clearly linked to patient outcome. Both patient mortality (Aiken, Clarke, Sloane, Sochalski, & Silber, 2002; Shekelle, 2013) and infection rate (Cimiotti, Aiken, Sloane, & Wu, 2012) inversely relate to nurse staff–to-patient ratio in acute care settings. Unfortunately, the nature of correctional health care delivery makes it difficult to apply specific staffing ratios. More work needs to be done on this important metric in the specialty.

- **Staffing mix** – the proportion of various licensed and unlicensed staff – has also been studied as it relates to patient safety and mortality. In particular, a greater proportion of registered nurse staffing correlates to fewer medication errors and lower fall rates in the acute care setting (Blegen & Vaughn, 1998). An increased proportion of licensed practical nurses in the staffing mix was linked to increased sepsis and mortality of trauma patients (Glance et al., 2012), while lower skill mixes (fewer RN staff) were linked with poorer patient outcomes in a retrospective study in Australian public hospitals (Twigg, Duffield, Bremner, Rapley, & Finn, 2012). Skill mix, then, is an important concern for patient safety in other settings, and more research may discern optimal skill mixes for correctional settings.

- **Shift work rotation** – continually changing staff shift assignments – means that workers' schedules are changed at regular intervals. Shift work is a necessary part of providing round-the-clock health care coverage and is a common part of most correctional settings. How an organization manages this shift work can also affect patient safety. Rotating staff around in different work shifts results in sleep disturbance and more accidents, as compared to permanent night shift workers in studies of industrial and telecommunication workers (Lundstrom et al., 2002). A study of Massachusetts nurses associated rotating shift work with frequent lapse of attention and increased reaction time resulting in increased error rates (D. R. Gold et al., 1992).

Studies in non-correctional health care settings link low nurse-patient ratios, lower staffing mix, and rotating shift work to poor patient outcomes (Lundstrom et al., 2002; Wachter, 2012). It is a fair assumption that this would be true in correctional settings as well. Even well-trained staff can be overworked and demoralized, thus leading to clinical error.

Cognitive Factors

The mental processes that a professional uses to make decisions and evaluate actions in delivering health care also contribute to patient safety or, conversely, clinical error. How people think, then, is an important component of a health care worker's contribution to safe patient care. Cognitive processes include determining where to focus attention in a clinical situation, activating and using knowledge in that situation, and dealing with both constraints and goals of the context of care delivery (Dekker, 2011).

Presented with a clinical situation, a practitioner must first decide what information, assessment findings, and clinical cues to gather and organize from a myriad of data available. Dekker (2011) suggests that clinicians mentally sort this information along a continuum, with some practitioners fixing early upon an interpretation of what is happening (called cognitive fixation) while others move from one explanation to another as new data emerges (called thematic vagabonding). He suggests a balanced approach that both fixes upon a probable explanation and enables consideration of other interpretations of the data. In a complex situation with much incongruent information, it can be helpful to bring in a new clinician with no vested interest in the current working diagnosis, who may interpret the constellation of data in a different configuration.

Application of knowledge to a clinical situation is another cognitive process that can affect a safe patient outcome. Here, too, a continuum exists between over-simplification into a cause-effect determination and over-analysis that leads to continual data collection and indecision. Seasoned practitioners develop pattern recognition based on knowledge and past experience. This pattern recognition, then, develops into cognitive shortcuts (called heuristics) that can speed the diagnosis of common conditions (Wachter, 2012). Although heuristics can be helpful, several biases of thought can derail pattern recognition and lead to error. Biases of greatest concern include availability, premature closure, framing effects, blind obedience, confirmation, representativeness, and sunk costs (Table 5.3). Clinicians must be aware of these potential cognitive errors and actively work to remove them from their habitual diagnostic reasoning processes.

In addition to the standard cognitive biases outlined in Table 5.3, correctional health care professionals must also struggle with the bias of cynicism so pervasive in the correctional culture. This cynicism is described as an "inappropriate distrust of prisoner patients...beyond the appropriate caution or skepticism that all professionals should have in their minds when confronted with a clinical puzzle"

Table 5.3 Cognitive Biases in Diagnostic Reasoning

Bias	Definition	Corrective Strategy
Availability	Determination based on ease of recalling past cases	Verify with legitimate statistics
Premature Closure	Relying too heavily on initial impressions	Reconsider determination in light of new data or a second opinion, consider extremes
Framing Effects	Being swayed by the description of the problem	Examine the case from alternative perspectives
Blind Obedience	Showing undue deference to authority or technology	Reconsider when authority is more remote; assess test accuracy
Confirmation	Seeking data to confirm, rather than refute, a favored hypothesis	Consciously seek both confirming and refuting data
Representativeness	Guided by typical features of a disease and missing atypical variants	Take into account typical and atypical findings before settling on a diagnosis
Sunk Costs	Difficulty considering alternative diagnoses once significant time, effort and resources have been invested in a particular diagnosis	Consider involving a second practitioner free of attachment to the favored diagnosis

Adapted from Nendaz & Perrier, 2012; Norman & Eva, 2010; Wachter, 2012

(Greifinger, 2013, p.3). This distrust of the incarcerated patient's health care request causes negative stereotyping and assumption of secondary motivations that lead the diagnostician away from a focus on the clinical condition. Thus, treatment delays, lapses in standard care, and needless deaths can result.

Finally, dealing with both constraints and goals in the context of care delivery is an area of cognitive work that contributes to the mental processing of a clinical situation. Clinicians rarely have the luxury of dealing with a single patient care situation at a time. Most are, instead, juggling the needs and concerns of a group of patients under their care. A simple example might be an emergency physician with four patients - a motorcycle trauma, an undetermined chest pain, a severed finger, and severe abdominal pain - who must determine priority of attention and the various diagnoses. The context of the clinical situation can complicate decision-making, such as the level of qualified staff available for various delegated procedures and the availability of the operating room or hospital beds for transfer.

Missed, Delayed, and Incorrect Diagnoses

Missed, delayed, or incorrect diagnoses are obvious patient safety concerns. A review of various studies of diagnostic error, including autopsy studies, patient surveys, and use of standardized patients, found diagnostic error rates of 10%-15% (Graber, 2013). A study of malpractice claims from the National Practitioner Data Bank found diagnostic error to be the most frequent and most costly of malpractice claims (Saber Tehrani et al., 2013). Many presume that incorrect diagnoses are most often related to rare or unusual conditions; however, case reviews indicate high numbers of missed diagnoses for such common conditions as strokes, childhood asthma, coronary artery disease, and malignancies (Graber, 2013). An estimated 40,000 to 80,000 patient deaths occur annually in hospitals due to diagnostic error (Hayward, 2002). No corresponding studies of patient deaths in the correctional setting were found, but it can be assumed that this is at least as prevalent.

Focusing specifically on cognitive errors that resulted in missed, delayed, or incorrect diagnoses, Graber and colleagues (2005) found four types of errors in a review of 100 cases from three academic medical centers. Their error categories are: 1) faulty knowledge; 2) faulty data gathering; 3) faulty information processing; and 4) faulty verification. These categories can help pinpoint weaknesses in the analytic process. The cognitive bias most often seen in these cases was premature closure - settling on a diagnosis too early (Graber, Franklin, & Gordon, 2005).

Faulty knowledge errors can result when a condition is rare or outside the diagnostician's specialty. With the wide array of conditions and challenging presentations in the patient community, medical staff entering the corrections specialty may have limited background in some conditions. Faulty data gathering may involve failure to perform standard screening procedures or collect typical information. Poor interactions with a challenging patient can limit full information. Information processing can be faulty if the clinician falls into any of the cognitive biases discussed in Table 5.3. It can also be hindered if a symptom is mistaken, such as referred pain. Finally, faulty verification can result from premature closure, a bias that leads to early diagnosis and lack of confirmative testing or evaluation. A clinician may fail to consult with an appropriate expert or be over-confident of their own diagnostic abilities (Graber et al., 2005).

System Errors that Affect Diagnostic Reasoning

System issues, particularly communication breakdowns, can also lead to diagnostic errors. Wachter (2012) suggests two primary categories of communication failures that affect diagnosis: those at the data gathering phase and those at the diagnostic verification phase. These two parts of the diagnostic process are most vulnerable to missing or incorrect information transmission. In an episodic and fragmented clinical system, such as some correctional settings, communication gaps in the diagnostic process can be plentiful.

Examples at the data gathering phase can include lack of complete information from a patient, missed phone calls or email responses, or assuming that a lack of response means that the information was dismissed as unimportant (Singh, Naik, Rao, & Petersen, 2008). A nurse performing sick call on the evening shift may leave a message for the physician that a patient has an unusual looking mole and assume that there will be follow-through. The physician may not receive the message and take no action. The nurse may perceive this lack of action to mean that the physician evaluated the mole and determined it to be benign.

Examples of communication breakdowns in the diagnostic verification phase involve missing or incorrect laboratory or diagnostic results. The lab technician can report critical values on the wrong patient or transcribe the critical lab value to the wrong patient's chart. In a system where there is a variety of on-call physicians, the ordering physician may not receive a critical value or be delayed in obtaining it, thus affecting the diagnostic process.

Reducing Diagnostic Error

Surprisingly, diagnostic error reduction has only recently been considered as a component of patient safety (Graber, Wachter, & Cassel, 2012). Thus, the research into ways to reduce diagnostic risk is minimal. Preliminary studies suggest the following actions to assist in improving diagnostic accuracy, some of which can be easily applied in the correctional setting.

- **Teaching cognitive skills.** Advances in the science of diagnostic decision-making means that even experienced practitioners need teaching in this area. Lack of practice or use results in decay of diagnostic skill (Weaver, Newman-

Toker, & Rosen, 2012). Continuing education of practitioners should include common biases and other sources of cognitive errors, along with multiple opportunities for active practice that involve actual patient presentations, recognition and response to diagnostic error, and use of decision support (Graber et al., 2005; Weaver et al., 2012).

- **Situation awareness and de-biasing.** Being mindful of the potential for cognitive bias that contributes to diagnostic error can reduce the potential for reasoning flaws (Graber, Kissam, et al., 2012). This can include using prospective hindsight, considering the potential consequences of an incorrect diagnosis. Situational awareness and prospective hindsight can reduce the chances of premature closure (Nendaz & Perrier, 2012).

- **Teaching patients.** Effectively communicating symptoms and complete health histories are important patient-focused components of accurate diagnoses. Several studies found that patient education in these areas improved diagnostic accuracy (McDonald et al., 2013). Once again, involving incarcerated patients in their own health care can improve patient safety, in this case through improved diagnostic accuracy.

- **Diagnostic checklists.** The use of checklists as mental prompts in other areas of patient safety concern has led to beginning work in the area of diagnostic checklists, both general and for specific high-risk diagnoses. The theory is that checklists help encourage more deliberative diagnostic thinking, thereby avoiding over-confidence and other cognitive biases such as premature closure and availability bias (Graber, Wachter, et al., 2012; Wachter, 2012). In one study, the use of a checklist reduced diagnostic error rates for electrocardiogram interpretation when used as a validation tool at the end of the diagnostic process (Sibbald, de Bruin, & van Merrienboer, 2013).

- **Decision support tools.** As digital information becomes more prevalent, decision support tools are being created to develop more comprehensive differential diagnoses. Traditional settings are testing differential diagnosis generators for widespread use (Bond et al., 2012). Alert systems that intervene for particular test results or symptom reduce diagnostic error and are increasingly included in electronic medical record systems (McDonald et al., 2013)

- **Trigger tools.** In line with decision support tools, trigger tools are most frequently used to generate notices when a treatment error may be present such as medication allergy or side effect. Promising use of triggers for diagnostic accuracy is also underway, such as a hospitalization within two weeks of a primary care visit triggering a re-evaluation of initial diagnosis (Singh et al., 2012).

- **System improvements.** Most system improvements under study to reduce diagnostic error involve the use of electronic documentation and communication. In addition to the use of decision support and triggering tools, electronic medical record systems are reducing communication gaps through prompts, tests tracking, and rapid access to diagnostic results both onsite and by mobile device (Schiff & Bates, 2010). As electronic medical record systems increase in the correctional setting, these system improvements become possible for reducing diagnostic errors in practice.

- **Reflection.** Health care professional education literature has also extensively studied mindful practice as it relates to diagnostic accuracy (Mann, Gordon, & MacLeod, 2009). Reflection in clinical practice is a cognitive process of thinking about our thinking to develop a greater understanding of ourselves and the situation. It can be engaged at any time in the diagnostic continuum, and helps the practitioner to make sense of a situation and intentionally learn from it (Sandars, 2009).

One of the most popular models for reflection describes a process involving noticing, processing, and altering action (Sandars, 2009). Noticing is a metacognitive skill of internal awareness of thought processes. This involves a deliberate and non-judgmental awareness of immediate thoughts and emotions. Noticing is followed by processing – developing an understanding of self and situation. The final component of reflection – altering action – is then a result of noticing and processing the experience.

Noticing, processing and altering action can take place during or after a diagnostic event. Reflection-in-action

"An inmate signed up for Nurse Sick Call stating that he had "lost sight in my left eye"; when he was seen by the sick call nurse, he told her "my sight is messed up – I can't see very well". Without further assessment, the nurse referred the inmate to Optometry Clinic for evaluation of his complaint of "decreased vision". The inmate was seen by the optometrist two weeks following the Sick Call visit. The optometrist examination revealed a detached retina. The inmate was immediately referred for ophthalmology evaluation, but it was too late to repair the detached retina and the inmate lost 50% vision in his left eye. The inmate subsequently sued and was compensated for his loss of vision. Reflection in action may have changed the course of this nursing encounter"
– Sue Smith, MSN, RN, CCHP-RN, Correctional Nurse Educator, Columbus, OH

requires intentionally slowing down the diagnostic process to accommodate a more deliberative approach. In fact, specifically asking the question "Could this be something else?" in the midst of the diagnostic process can increase more deliberative analysis (Graber, et al., 2012). Reflection-on-action, on the other hand, is a retrospective look at a prior experience to gain personal insight and learning from the experience. In this case, noticing and processing a past experience then leads to altering future action.

Clinicians most often naturally engage in reflection during training for the profession and when a particularly challenging or perplexing clinical puzzle presents itself. Intentional reflection correlates to the development of expertise in a particular area of practice, such as diagnostic accuracy (Mamede & Schmidt, 2004). Reflection can mitigate against predominant use of pattern recognition as the standard diagnostic process, fraught with all the inherent cognitive biases. A reflective practitioner frames and reframes a problem, considers a broad range of factors before settling on a diagnosis, and is willing to remain uncertain for a longer period of time while considering options (Mamede et al., 2007). Besides metacognitive engagement in the midst of the diagnostic process, a reflective practitioner reflectively reviews past decisions, looking for learning experiences and patterns in the diagnostic presentation, thus adjusting thought processes for future experiences.

Unfortunately, reflection tends to decrease with experience (Mamede & Schmidt, 2005). This decline can be troubling in an ever-changing and advancing health care system. Practitioners must be ever mindful of over-emphasis on pattern recognition as practice experience develops. This can be especially true in a specialty such as corrections, where practitioners must keep abreast of a wide array of conditions and treatments to meet the primary care needs of the patient population. Encouraging reflective practice can decrease cognitive skill decay and encourage balanced diagnostic reasoning practices.

The following methods for encouraging reflective practice have application in the correctional clinical setting.

- **A Culture of reflection.** An organizational culture that appreciates openness and learning encourages and nurtures reflective practice. As with establishing a Just Culture, described in Chapter 2, establishing a culture of reflection requires effort, including attention to barriers to reflection-in-action (such as a time-pressed environment that does not allow for a thoughtful review of alternatives) or barriers to reflection-on-practice (such as a lack of openness to learning from errors or even acknowledging that errors can happen).

- **Peer review reflection.** Feedback improves diagnostic expertise and error awareness (Graber, Kissam, et al., 2012). Peer review, a standard in most medical practices, can be an opportunity for enhanced peer collaboration and reflection on a particular clinical case. Here, too, clinicians must be willing to openly explore possible errors in diagnostic reasoning and look for opportunities to improve.

- **Small group reflection.** Small group processes can stimulate reflection (Mann et al., 2009). Case presentations in a "grand rounds" approach or even during regular team meetings can prompt reflection while encouraging learning for both the diagnostician and others in the care team. In like manner, morbidity and mortality reviews provide opportunity for reflection on diagnostic practice.

Summary

Throughout the continuum of practice, health care workers have an opportunity to improve patient safety by developing and maintaining clinical competency. Internal and external factors can affect competency in the active context of care delivery, and organizations should adapt practices accordingly to reduce clinical error. Health care workers must be aware of their own biopsychosocial well-being and take steps to reduce physical and compassion fatigue or work stress, when possible. This includes actively monitoring general health and well-being to determine if disease or medical treatment may be impairing clear thinking and dexterity. Individual workers and their teammates also have a responsibility to be aware of potential substance use issues. Organizations, however, have a primary responsibility for attending to external factors such as staffing ratios, staffing mixes, and shift work – all factors that affect an employee's ability to deliver safe patient care.

Diagnostic error is a new area of patient safety investigation, with up to 15% of medical diagnoses found to be incorrect. How diagnosticians process data to make clinical decisions and the factors affecting decision-making is currently under investigation. Although research is presently sparse, clinicians and organizations can apply cognitive skill education and decision-making tools to assist diagnosticians to make accurate medical diagnoses.

References

Adams, R.E., Boscarino, J.A., & Figley, C.R. (2006). Compassion fatigue and psychological distress among social workers: A validation study. *The American Journal of Orthopsychiatry, 76*(1), 103–108. doi:10.1037/0002-9432.76.1.103

Aiken, L.H., Clarke, S.P., Sloane, D.M., Sochalski, J., & Silber, J.H. (2002). Hospital nurse staffing and patient mortality, nurse burnout, and job dissatisfaction. *JAMA: The Journal of the American Medical Association, 288*(16), 1987–1993.

American College of Healthcare Executives. (2013). Impaired healthcare executives. *Healthcare Executive, 28*(3), 118–119.

American Correctional Health Services Association (ACHSA). *Mission and ethics statement.* Retrieved from http://www.achsa.org/mission-ethics-statement/

American Medical Association (AMA). (2011). *American Medical Association policies related to physician health.* Retrieved from http://www.ama-assn.org/resources/doc/physician-health/policies-physician-health.pdf

American Nurses Association (ANA). (1984). Addictions and psychological dysfunctions in nursing: The profession's response to the problem. *American Nurses Association Publications*, (PMH-6), i–iv, 1–36.

American Nurses Association (ANA). (2001). *Code of ethics for nurses with interpretive statements.* Silver Springs, MD: American Nurses Association. Retrieved from http://www.nursingworld.org/MainMenuCategories/EthicsStandards/CodeofEthicsforNurses/Code-of-Ethics.pdf

American Nurses Association (ANA). (2006, December 8). *Assuring patient safety: Registered nurses' responsibility in all roles and settings to guard against working when fatigued.* Retrieved from http://www.nursingworld.org/MainMenuCategories/Policy-Advocacy/Positions-and-Resolutions/ANAPositionStatements/Position-Statements-Alphabetically/Copy-of-AssuringPatientSafety-1.pdf

Amin, M.M., Graber, M., Ahmad, K., Manta, D., Hossain, S., Belisova, Z., … Gold, A.R. (2012). The effects of a mid-day nap on the neurocognitive performance of first-year medical residents: A controlled interventional pilot study. *Academic Medicine: Journal of the Association of American Medical Colleges, 87*(10), 1428–1433. doi:10.1097/ACM.0b013e3182676b37

Argentero, P. & Setti, I. (2011). Engagement and vicarious traumatization in rescue workers. *International Archives of Occupational and Environmental Health, 84*(1), 67–75. doi:10.1007/s00420-010-0601-8

Baldisseri, M.R. (2007). Impaired healthcare professional. *Critical Care Medicine, 35*(Suppl), S106–S116. doi:10.1097/01.CCM.0000252918.87746.96

Benton, J.H. & Flynn, J. (2013). Identifying and minimizing risk exposures affecting nursing practice to enhance patient safety. *Journal of Nursing Regulation, 3*(4), 4–9.

Berner, E.S. & Graber, M.L. (2008). Overconfidence as a cause of diagnostic error in medicine. *The American Journal of Medicine, 121*(5 Suppl), S2–23. doi:10.1016/j.amjmed.2008.01.001

Blegen, M.A. & Vaughn, T. (1998). A multisite study of nurse staffing and patient occurrences. *Nursing Economic$, 16*(4), 196–203.

Blum, R. H., Raemer, D. B., Carroll, J. S., Dufresne, R. L., & Cooper, J. B. (2005). A method for measuring the effectiveness of simulation-based team training for improving communication skills. *Anesthesia and Analgesia, 100*(5), 1375–1380. doi:10.1213/01.ANE.0000148058.64834.80

Bohne, P. & Peruzzi, W. (2010). A just culture supports patient safety. *Trustee: The Journal for Hospital Governing Boards, 63*(4), 32–3.

Bond, W.F., Schwartz, L.M., Weaver, K.R., Levick, D., Giuliano, M., & Graber, M.L. (2012). Differential diagnosis generators: An evaluation of currently available computer programs. *Journal of General Internal Medicine, 27*(2), 213–219. doi:10.1007/s11606-011-1804-8

Broscio, M.A. (2013). Behavioral interviewing: Back to the future. *Healthcare Executive*, (July/Aug), 56–57.

Bryant, C., Fairbrother, G., & Fenton, P. (2000). The relative influence of personal and workplace descriptors on stress. *British Journal of Nursing, 9*(13), 876–880.

Cimiotti, J.P., Aiken, L.H., Sloane, D.M., & Wu, E.S. (2012). Nurse staffing, burnout, and health care-associated infection. *American Journal of Infection Control, 40*(6), 486–490. doi:10.1016/j.ajic.2012.02.029

Cook, D.A., Erwin, P.J., & Triola, M.M. (2010). Computerized virtual patients in health professions education: A systematic review and meta-analysis. *Academic Medicine: Journal of the Association of American Medical Colleges, 85*(10), 1589–1602. doi:10.1097/ACM.0b013e3181edfe13

Croskerry, P. (2005). Diagnostic failure: A cognitive and affective approach. In K. Henriksen, J. B. Battles, E.S. Marks, & D.I. Lewin (Eds.), *Advances in Patient Safety: From Research to Implementation (Volume 2: Concepts and Methodology)*. Rockville, MD: Agency for Healthcare Research and Quality (US). Retrieved from http://www.ncbi.nlm.nih.gov/books/NBK20487/

Croskerry, P. (2009a). A universal model of diagnostic reasoning. *Academic Medicine: Journal of the Association of American Medical Colleges, 84*(8), 1022–1028. doi:10.1097/ACM.0b013e3181ace703

Croskerry, P. (2009b). Clinical cognition and diagnostic error: Applications of a dual process model of reasoning. *Advances in Health Sciences Education: Theory and Practice, 14 Suppl 1*, 27–35. doi:10.1007/s10459-009-9182-2

Dekker, S. (2011). *Patient safety: A human factors approach*. Boca Raton, FL: CRC Press.

Diaz, D. A., Panosky, D. M., & Shelton, D. (2014). Simulation: Introduction to correctional nursing in a prison setting. *Journal of Correctional Health Care, 20*(3), 240-248, doi:10.1177/1078345814532324

Dunkley, J. & Whelan, T.A. (2006). Vicarious traumatisation: Current status and future directions. *British Journal of Guidance & Counselling, 34*(1), 107–116. doi:10.1080/03069880500483166

Ely, J.W., Graber, M.L., & Croskerry, P. (2011). Checklists to reduce diagnostic errors. *Academic Medicine: Journal of the Association of American Medical Colleges, 86*(3), 307–313. doi:10.1097/ACM.0b013e31820824cd

Emanuel, L., Berwick, D., Conway, J., Combes, J., Hatlie, M., Leape, L., ... Walton, M. (2008). What exactly is patient safety. *Advances in Patient Safety: New Directions and Alternative Approaches, 1*. Retrieved from http://ahrq.hhs.gov/downloads/pub/advances2/vol1/Advances-Emanuel-Berwick_110.pdf

Gaba, D.M. & Howard, S.K. (2002). Fatigue among clinicians and the safety of patients. *New England Journal of Medicine, 347*(16), 1249–1255.

Gilbert, G.L., Cheung, P.Y., & Kerridge, I.B. (2009). Infection control, ethics and accountability. *Medical Journal of Australia, 190*(12), 696–698.

Glance, L.G., Dick, A.W., Osler, T.M., Mukamel, D.B., Li, Y., & Stone, P.W. (2012). The association between nurse staffing and hospital outcomes in injured patients. *BMC Health Services Research, 12*, 247. doi:10.1186/1472-6963-12-247

Gold, D.R., Rogacz, S., Bock, N., Tosteson, T.D., Baum, T.M., Speizer, F.E., & Czeisler, C.A. (1992). Rotating shift work, sleep, and accidents related to sleepiness in hospital nurses. *American Journal of Public Health, 82*(7), 1011–1014.

Gold, K.B. & Teitelbaum, M.D. (2010). Physicians impaired by substance abuse disorders. *The Journal of Global Drug Policy and Practice.* Retrieved from http://globaldrugpolicy.info/Issues/Vol%202%20Issue%202/Physicians%20Impaired%20by%20Substance%20Abuse%20Disorders.pdf

Gottlieb, B.H., Kelloway, E.K., & Martin-Matthews, A. (1996). Predictors of work-family conflict, stress, and job satisfaction among nurses. *Revue Canadienne de Recherche En Sciences Infirmières (The Canadian Journal of Nursing Research), 28*(2), 99–117.

Graber, M.L. (2013). The incidence of diagnostic error in medicine. *BMJ Quality & Safety, 22 Suppl 2*, ii21–ii27. doi:10.1136/bmjqs-2012-001615

Graber, M.L., Franklin, N., & Gordon, R. (2005). Diagnostic error in internal medicine. *Archives of Internal Medicine, 165*(13), 1493–1499. doi:10.1001/archinte.165.13.1493

Graber, M.L., Kissam, S., Payne, V.L., Meyer, A.N.D., Sorensen, A., Lenfestey, N., ... Singh, H. (2012). Cognitive interventions to reduce diagnostic error: A narrative review. *BMJ Quality & Safety, 21*(7), 535–557. doi:10.1136/bmjqs-2011-000149

Graber, M.L., Wachter, R.M., & Cassel, C.K. (2012). Bringing diagnosis into the quality and safety equations. *JAMA: The Journal of the American Medical Association, 308*(12), 1211–1212. doi:10.1001/2012.jama.11913

Greifinger, R. B. (2013). The acid bath of cynicism. *Correctional Law Reporter, June/July*, 3,14,16.

Hayward, R.A. (2002). Counting deaths due to medical errors. *JAMA: The Journal of the American Medical Association, 288*(19), 2404–2405; author reply 2405.

Hoffman, P. (2009). Health care legal concepts. In R. Carroll, (Ed.), *Risk management handbook for health care organizations* (Student ed., pp. 115–157). San Francisco, CA: Jossey-Bass.

Jennings, B.M. (2008). Work stress and burnout among nurses: Role of the work environment and working conditions. In R.G. Hughes (Ed.), *Patient safety and quality: An evidence-based handbook for nurses*. Rockville (MD): Agency for Healthcare Research and Quality (US). Retrieved from http://www.ncbi.nlm. nih.gov/books/NBK2668/

Kunyk, D. (2013). Substance use disorders among registered nurses: Prevalence, risks and perceptions in a disciplinary jurisdiction. *Journal of Nursing Management*. doi:10.1111/jonm.12081

Lovato, N. & Lack, L. (2010). The effects of napping on cognitive functioning. *Progress in Brain Research, 185*, 155–166. doi:10.1016/B978-0-444-53702-7.00009-9

Lundstrom, T., Pugliese, G., Bartley, J., Cox, J., & Guither, C. (2002). Organizational and environmental factors that affect worker health and safety and patient outcomes. *American Journal of Infection Control, 30*(2), 93–106.

Mamede, S. & Schmidt, H.G. (2004). The structure of reflective practice in medicine. *Medical Education, 38*(12), 1302–1308. doi:10.1111/j.1365-2929.2004.01917.x

Mamede, S., & Schmidt, H. G. (2005). Correlates of reflective practice in medicine. *Advances in Health Sciences Education: Theory and Practice, 10*(4), 327–337. doi:10.1007/s10459-005-5066-2

Mamede, S., Schmidt, H.G., & Rikers, R. (2007). Diagnostic errors and reflective practice in medicine. *Journal of Evaluation in Clinical Practice, 13*(1), 138–145. doi:10.1111/j.1365-2753.2006.00638.x

Mann, K., Gordon, J., & MacLeod, A. (2009). Reflection and reflective practice in health professions education: A systematic review. *Advances in Health Sciences Education: Theory and Practice, 14*(4), 595–621. doi:10.1007/s10459-007-9090-2

Marx, D. (2001). *Patient safety and the "Just Culture": A primer for health care executives*. New York, NY: Columbia University. Retrieved from http://www. safer.healthcare.ucla.edu/safer/archive/ahrq/FinalPrimerDoc.pdf

McDonald, K.M., Matesic, B., Contopoulos-Ioannidis, D.G., Lonhart, J., Schmidt, E., Pineda, N., & Ioannidis, J.P.A. (2013). Patient safety strategies targeted at diagnostic errors: A systematic review. *Annals of Internal Medicine, 158*(5 Pt 2), 381–389. doi:10.7326/0003-4819-158-5-201303051-00004

McGaghie, W.C., Issenberg, S.B., Cohen, E.R., Barsuk, J.H., & Wayne, D.B. (2011). Does simulation-based medical education with deliberate practice yield better results than traditional clinical education? A meta-analytic comparative review of the evidence. *Academic Medicine: Journal of the Association of American Medical Colleges, 86*(6), 706–711. doi:10.1097/ACM.0b013e318217e119

Milner, C.E. & Cote, K.A. (2009). Benefits of napping in healthy adults: Impact of nap length, time of day, age, and experience with napping. *Journal of Sleep Research, 18*(2), 272–281. doi:10.1111/j.1365-2869.2008.00718.x

Munger, T. (2013). *When caring for perpetrators becomes a sentence: Recognizing vicarious trauma*. Unpublished manuscript.

Nendaz, M. & Perrier, A. (2012). Diagnostic errors and flaws in clinical reasoning: Mechanisms and prevention in practice. *Swiss Medical Weekly, 142,* w13706. doi:10.4414/smw.2012.13706

Norman, G.R. & Eva, K.W. (2010). Diagnostic error and clinical reasoning. *Medical Education, 44*(1), 94–100. doi:10.1111/j.1365-2923.2009.03507.x

Pross, C. (2006). Burnout, vicarious traumatization and its prevention. *Torture: Quarterly Journal on Rehabilitation of Torture Victims and Prevention of Torture, 16*(1), 1–9.

Rogers, A.E. & Hughes, R.G. (2008). The effects of fatigue and sleepiness on nurse performance and patient safety. *Patient Safety and Quality: An Evidence-Based Handbook for Nurses,* 2–509.

Russell, K.A. (2012). Nurse practice acts guide and govern nursing practice. *Journal of Nursing Regulation, 3*(3), 36–42.

Saber Tehrani, A.S., Lee, H., Mathews, S.C., Shore, A., Makary, M.A., Pronovost, P.J., & Newman-Toker, D.E. (2013). 25-year summary of US malpractice claims for diagnostic errors 1986-2010: An analysis from the National Practitioner Data Bank. *BMJ Quality & Safety, 22*(8), 672–680. doi:10.1136/bmjqs-2012-001550

Sabo, B. (2011). Reflecting on the concept of compassion fatigue. *Online Journal of Issues in Nursing, 16*(1), 1. Retrieved from http://www.nursingworld.org/MainMenuCategories/ANAMarketplace/ANAPeriodicals/OJIN/TableofContents/Vol-16-2011/No1-Jan-2011/Concept-of-Compassion-Fatigue.html

Sandars, J. (2009). The use of reflection in medical education: AMEE Guide No. 44. *Medical Teacher, 31*(8), 685–695.

Schiff, G.D. & Bates, D.W. (2010). Can electronic clinical documentation help prevent diagnostic errors? *The New England Journal of Medicine, 362*(12), 1066–1069. doi:10.1056/NEJMp0911734

Schmidt, E.M., Goldhaber-Fiebert, S.N., Ho, L.A., & McDonald, K.M. (2013). *Use of simulation exercises in patient safety efforts*. Retrieved from http://www.ncbi.nlm.nih.gov/pubmedhealth/PMH0055922/

Schweitzer, P.K., Randazzo, A.C., Stone, K., Erman, M., & Walsh, J.K. (2006). Laboratory and field studies of naps and caffeine as practical countermeasures for sleep-wake problems associated with night work. *Sleep, 29*(1), 39–50.

Shekelle, P.G. (2013). Nurse-patient ratios as a patient safety strategy: A systematic review. *Annals of Internal Medicine, 158*(5 Pt 2), 404–409. doi:10.7326/0003-4819-158-5-201303051-00007

Shelton, D., Weiskopf, C., & Nicholson, M. (2010). Correctional nursing competency development in the Connecticut Correctional Managed Health Care Program. *Journal of Correctional Health Care, 16*(4), 299–309. doi:10.1177/1078345810378498

Sibbald, M., de Bruin, A.B.H., & van Merrienboer, J.J.G. (2013). Checklists improve experts' diagnostic decisions. *Medical Education, 47*(3), 301–308. doi:10.1111/medu.12080

Singh, H., Giardina, T.D., Forjuoh, S.N., Reis, M.D., Kosmach, S., Khan, M.M., & Thomas, E.J. (2012). Electronic health record-based surveillance of diagnostic errors in primary care. *BMJ Quality & Safety, 21*(2), 93–100. doi:10.1136/bmjqs-2011-000304

Singh, H., Naik, A.D., Rao, R., & Petersen, L.A. (2008). Reducing diagnostic errors through effective communication: Harnessing the power of information technology. *Journal of General Internal Medicine, 23*(4), 489–494. doi:10.1007/s11606-007-0393-z

Society of Correctional Physicians (SCP). (n.d.) *SCP code of ethics*. Retrieved from http://societyofcorrectionalphysicians.org/resources/code-of-ethics

Spath, P. (2011). *Error reduction in health care a systems approach to improving patient safety*. San Francisco, CA: Jossey-Bass. Retrieved from http://site.ebrary.com/id/10452931

Stern, M.F., Greifinger, R.B., & Mellow, J. (2010). Patient safety: Moving the bar in prison health care standards. *American Journal of Public Health, 100*(11), 2103.

The Joint Commission (TJC). (2005). *The Joint Commission guide to improving staff communication*. Oakbrook Terrace, IL: Joint Commission Resources.

The Joint Commission (TJC). (2012). New alert warns of risks associated with health care worker fatigue. *Joint Commission Perspectives, 32*(3). Retrieved from http://www.ingentaconnect.com/content/jcaho/jcp/2012/00000032/00000003/art00006

Thomas, C.M. & Siela, D. (2011). The impaired nurse: Would you know what to do if you suspected substance abuse? *American Nurse Today, 6*(8). Retrieved from http://www.americannursetoday.com/article.aspx?id=8114&fid=8078

Trinkoff, A.M., Geiger-Brown, J.M., Caruso, C.C., Lipscomb, J.A., Johantgen, M., Nelson, A.L., ... Selby, V.L. (2008). Personal safety for nurses. In R.G. Hughes (Ed.), *Patient safety and quality: An evidence-based handbook for nurses*. Rockville, MD: Agency for Healthcare Research and Quality (US). Retrieved from http://www.ncbi.nlm.nih.gov/books/NBK2661/

Twigg, D., Duffield, C., Bremner, A., Rapley, P., & Finn, J. (2012). Impact of skill mix variations on patient outcomes following implementation of nursing hours per patient day staffing: A retrospective study. *Journal of Advanced Nursing, 68*(12), 2710–2718. doi:10.1111/j.1365-2648.2012.05971.x

Wachter, R.M. (2012). Understanding patient safety (2nd ed.). New York, NY: Mcgraw-Hill.

Weaver, S.J., Newman-Toker, D.E., & Rosen, M.A. (2012). Reducing cognitive skill decay and diagnostic error: Theory-based practices for continuing education in health care. *The Journal of Continuing Education in the Health Professions, 32*(4), 269–278. doi:10.1002/chp.21155

World Medical Association (WMA). (2006, January 10). *WMA International Code of Medical Ethics*. Retrieved January 24, 2014, from http://www.wma.net/en/30publications/10policies/c8/index.html

Index

54608917R00088

Made in the USA
Middletown, DE
05 December 2017